# Pearley's Pearls

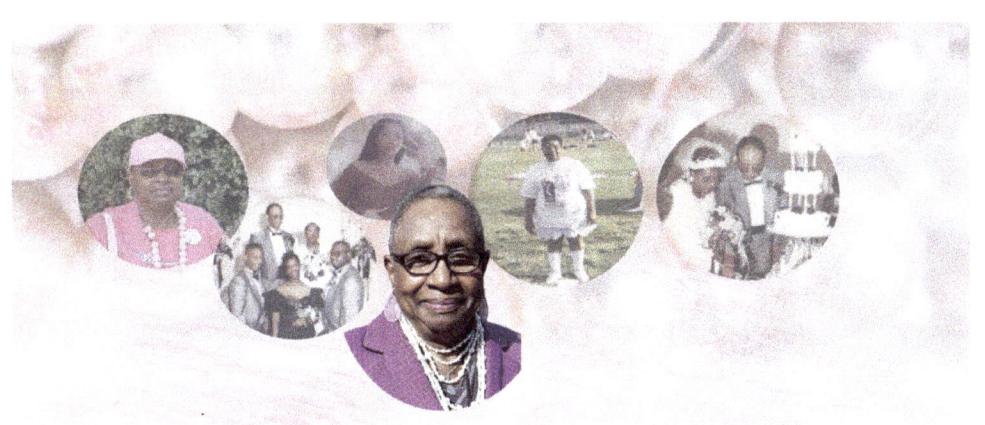

# Pearley's Pearls
## Wisdom From My Journey Through Life

PEARLEY LONG YELVERTON

# DEDICATION

All praise and thanksgiving to **God** from whom all blessings flow. How excellent is thou name in all the earth. All I am and all that I hope to be, I owe it all to **JESUS.** You rebooted, optimized, energized and increased my faith, and broadened my knowledge.

This book is dedicated to my parents, Mr. **Joe** and Mrs. **Sallie** Long.

To my late husband, **Clarence**, "Pee Wee," your memories are etched on my heart, and you shaped me into the woman I am today.

To My Children:

- **Clarence Jr.**, in heaven, you are missed.
- **Grear,** thank you for stepping in your Daddy's shoes and your commitment to our family.
- **Bernard**, you are my private eye, prayer partner, and personal caregiver, thank you for honoring me as a Proverbs 31 Woman.
- **Nikki**, my mover and team captain: when my faith dwindles, you always speak life into me.
- My beloved Granddaughter, **Jordyn**, you are my greatest cheerleader.

This book is my legacy, and I give you my best.

All my love,

Pearley

# ACKNOWLEDGEMENTS

To my loving family, thank you for your support in difficult times.

- **James A. Long, Sr**.
- **Ernest Long, Sr.**
- **Carolyn L. Bane, Ph.D**. and **Bane**
- **Beverly L. Joseph, Ph.D**. and **Michael**
- Cousin **Linda Bailey and George**
- Niece **Valencia Williams**
- **My late Aunt Thelma, Dr. Daphne** and the **Wiggins Family**
- **Robert and Geraldine King** and **my extended Yelverton Family**

There have been many who have traveled with me in and out of season, and I am truly grateful; however, I would be remiss not to mention:

- **Rev. Dr. Prince R. Rivers and Family**
- **Rev. Dr. Kenneth R. Hammond and Family**
- **Mother Berneice Kinsbury and Family**
- **Rev. Jessie McLain**
- **Professor Grover and Audrey Wilson**
- **Saravette Paige and Family and Francis Joyner**
- **Rev. Leroy and Pat Pegram**
- **Carver and Louise Joyner**

- Juliet Black and Family
- Rev. Rana and Gary Davis and Family
- Union Baptist and Greater St. Paul Church Families and B.F. Person Class of 1964
- Charlotte Purvis
- Sandra Albright
- Rev. Dexter Wright

To the **readers**, thank you for your dedication.

A very special thanks to **Penda L. James, Scribe Coach**, for all your prayers, knowledge, dedication to publishing my book, and encouragement in getting this done. I will be forever grateful.

Someone asked why I thanked so many people. I said, "It took the whole village to raise the child, and it was this village that walked with me on this journey."

# INTRODUCTION
## PEARLS OF WISDOM

Buckle your seatbelt and come ride with me through my life. This is my journey of tests, trials, tragedies, triumphs, and restoration. Good, bad, and ugly experiences don't last forever, even if they seem to stick around. I hope you find comfort in my story not just for the moment, but as a constant reminder that life is only a test drive. Eventually, the wheels will turn and there will be a new beginning.

I believe a time will come for every woman to slow down, turn off her cell phone, and close her laptop. This is that time for you. I want you to become familiar with the rocky road conditions that I had to navigate around, so that you can avoid my pitfalls. I'll teach you how to be cautious on the highway of life and how to "let the praise time begin," as you recognize that our God is always good.

Become familiar with the words "Grace" and "Mercy," because they have been present throughout my life. While I was trying to avoid potholes in the road, my Savior, Jesus Christ, was transforming my soul through an intricate reconstruction of my faith and of my physical body.

## An Intricate Reconstruction

At this season in my life, as I am sending *Pearley's Pearls* out to the world, I think back to my childhood on Dyking Road. In my childhood, I experienced several tragedies, and as an adult, multiple medical prognoses. I embrace the gift of life and count my blessings every single day.

I have survived breast cancer and have lived with epilepsy, both in remission for many years. I celebrate my life with these conditions, and my hopes of spreading awareness guide me daily. Each day presents new challenges, but I am thankful to God for the support of friends, family, and caregivers. I will stand at the "pulpit of praise," as I share about God developing my faith like a photographer in a dark room, and Him delivering me from the prison walls of Epilepsy.

The time it took me to recover from those setbacks was lengthy and felt overwhelming; yet God was with me. I ran on empty through life's construction sites, riding by faith, while God took the wheel from me.

I give God all of the praise because He has truly blessed me to live with epilepsy for many years. Epilepsy is widely known but barely understood. Those of us who live with epilepsy are human, and we deserve respect. I am so happy for continued research and the hope for a cure. There are new medications, and we as epilepsy survivors now have a voice in our healthcare. Christ is the hope of Glory to help us through it.

## A Spiritual Ride

I want to describe a spiritual experience that may sound familiar to you. Have you ever been riding along and out of nowhere had car trouble? In Kittrell, North Carolina, where I am from, we have a lot of rocky roads in the country. One day, I had a vision where I felt like I was driving on one of those roads. My spiritual engine was shutting down. One by one, my systems were stopping, and everything from my medical system, my emotional system and my physical system were not functioning. Like a car would, I needed an engine specialist to diagnose, service and repair me.

For me, that specialist was Jesus. In my vision, I saw myself driving one morning. I was scanning the streets outside of the window looking for a place to fill up my gas tank. The gas light was on, and I had a wallet full of gas cards, but no gas stations were nearby. When I finally started running on empty, I called Triple A (AAA). They answered the call but kept me on hold. I got annoyed hearing the recording, "Thank you for waiting. Your call is important to us and will be answered in the order it was received." If that recording had played one more time, I was going to scream!

I became so emotional that I drifted over to a safe spot to catch my breath. Then I pulled over and shut down the roadside, blocking traffic behind me.

Can you imagine the impatient people behind me? They were pulling their cars around me laying on their car horns, shouting, "Move out of the way, lady."

I sat there, feeling overwhelmed and in my emotions for a few minutes. After what felt like forever, I heard a voice say, "Ma'am, I have you on a direct line with the Specialist."

That news calmed me. I opened my heart and allowed Jesus to take the wheel. I slid over, and He increased my faith by flushing everything toxic from my spiritual radiator. Piece by piece, I was healed. So much time had passed, so much had happened, I thought I would never finish my journey.

By the time the Specialist arrived, it felt so dark around me. I felt Him reassembling my transmission and resetting my mirrors. When I turned the key, my engine that had stalled restarted. My old windshield wipers were exchanged for new ones, and my slate was wiped clean. I flicked my lights on feeling fully restored. The Specialist helped me get back up and running!

**Continuing My Journey**

Thankfully, the idea of writing a book wouldn't let me go. I started in 2017, and I knew I had to write to set in motion a true reformation of faith for others. While writing, I had so many hurdles to jump over. It seemed like once I was over one hurdle, I fell downhill and had to get back in position. It happened so much that I wasn't sure I wanted to write anymore. The gaps and pauses set me back, but when I would write late at night, my granddaughter, Jordyn, would jump off of my bed to keep me awake. She would say, "Grandma, look at me. I am keeping you awake so you won't make a mistake." Those precious moments stay with me even though she is much older now.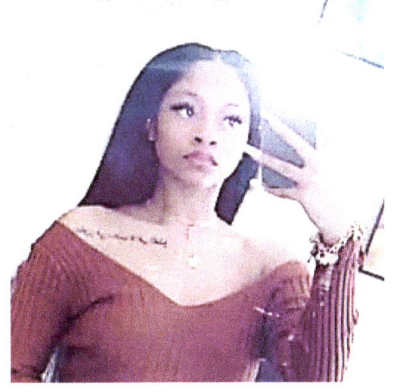

I broke my dominant hand in 2019 and couldn't write to finish my book. That break led me to being hospitalized for surgery. God sent people to be my anointed helping hands, and I am grateful for Domita White, Hazel Holmes, Reggie and Michelle Reavis, Ruby Singletary, Bernice Harris, and Rev. and Mrs. Amos Glover. They helped me care for myself in so many personal ways, God reminded me again that He was with me.

I had physical therapy and injections in my thumb during 2020. Then, when the COVID-19 shutdown was announced, tears rolled down my cheeks as I exchanged the pain of my hand for the pain of another, COVID-19. My book was put on hold, again.

During the Pandemic, I needed to find something to do other than watch COVID-19 casualty numbers rise. God taught me to be still and find joy and peace through writing. The shutdown inspired me to do something positive. I began writing again and God restored my soul. My writing helped me make a right turn into the path of Grace and Mercy which took over the wheels and drove me through a fast line of traffic in the complex lessons of COVID-19.

Life has taken me in many directions. I am nearing my yellow brick road toward my home, just like Dorothy in the Wizard of Oz. These *Pearley's Pearls* of wisdom that I am sharing will help you stay on your road of faith.

# CONTENTS

# DYKING ROAD

*I praise Him for I am fearfully and wonderfully made; marvelous are thy works; my soul knows this right well."*
Psalm 139:14

God laid the path for me when I was formed in my Mother's womb. Like people stand on the Psalms in the Bible, I stand on the backs of my parents, Joe and Sallie Long. They are my foundational tools and are forever present in my life. One thing I learned from my parents is that marriage is not a dictatorship, but a partnership of love, respect, giving and receiving. I can affirm that my most memorable times in life were back on the farm with my family.

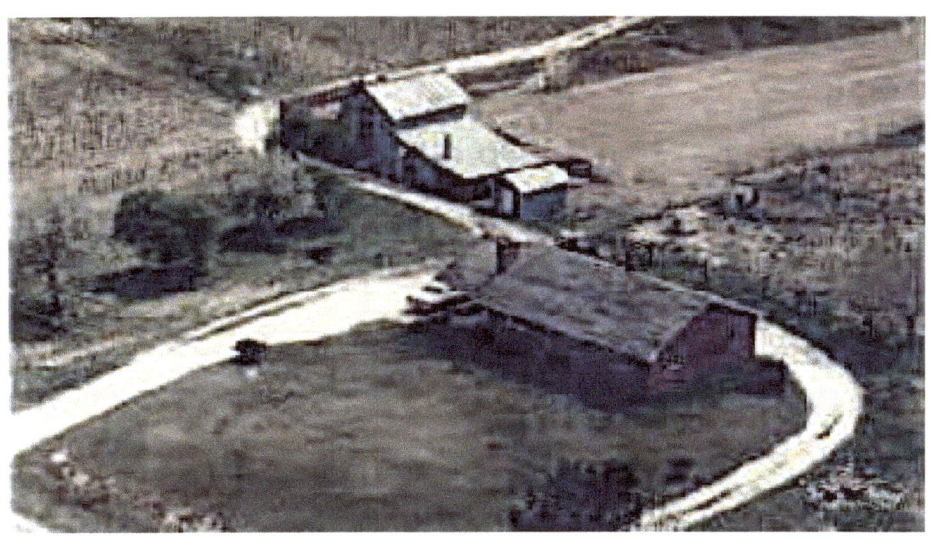

I was born in 1946, and I was reared on Dyking Road in Kittrell, North Carolina. My parents were strict, and I didn't have the same privileges as my younger sisters. Entering the city, there was a sign that said, "Welcome to Kittrell." If you blinked you'd see another one saying, "Come Back Soon."

The whole village raised me and nurtured me early. Children were seen, not heard, and everyone tended to their own business. What happened at home stayed at home. We didn't share our home life with anyone outside of our family.

Our mornings began by landing on our feet and hitting the floor moving toward the kitchen for a bowl of Mother's hot oatmeal. She used to say with assurance, "This is the healthy way to start a new day." Because of her, I still believe being a homemaker is the greatest profession one can hold.

Family was a homemade product of an old-fashioned mom with strong morals and values. Mother would fry up chicken and make gravy for her golden brown biscuits. We ate whatever we raised. I can still see the chickens running across the yard, the cattle and the pigs in our barn. We milked the cows and drank fresh milk daily.

We loved eating Mother's biscuits fresh out of the oven. Before we could eat, Mother would have a long prayer telling Jesus everything. By the time she was finished, the food would be cold.

Daddy had a truck, and he would ride down Main Street of Louisburg, North Carolina ringing his bell saying, "Joe's Garden." For money, he sold our extra pigs, corn, tomatoes, yellow squash, butter beans, string beans, collard greens, turnip greens and a whole lot more. We canned and preserved pickles and made jelly, which we stored in glass jars. Those were the good days on Dyking Road.

Not only did I work on the farm, but my volunteering skills also began at an early age; we didn't have a lot of activities away from the Long family campus, other than church. My great grandfather, Andrew Jackson Green, was the founder of Concord Baptist Church. Among my four limited childhood activities were attending Haywood Baptist; Baptist Training Union (BTU); Sunday School at Concord Baptist, where my writing talents were awakened; and the 4-H club, whose pledge I memorized as a child. That pledge remains in my heart to this day.

Daddy was the greatest farmer in Franklin County. Many sharecroppers looked to him as a mentor. He took care of his sixty-two acres and was very proud of that. Daddy and Mother beat the odds; they were able to purchase property and build a home for us from the ground up. We were Franklin County tax payees. We had so much fun on the farm, we didn't even realize we were poor.

When my brother, Ernest, and his bride Barbara decided to get married in 1959, Daddy insisted that they have their dream wedding on his property. It was a beautiful Saturday afternoon and Rev. Blaylock officiated. My brother's wedding was the talk of the country roads.

## Foundational Tools

We had a Saturday night tradition where everyone took turns climbing into a big tin tub to take a bath. Today most people have their own tub and shower, but we didn't have that luxury.

Sunday morning worship was the highlight of our week. We put on our Sunday best for church. Mother's straightening comb was always out, yet she would wait until Sunday morning to straighten our hair. I remember the feeling of my ear frying, or the sound of the straightening comb on her finger, whichever she hit first.

Back then, Mother kept my hair straight. Today in the 21st century, we have hot combs, flat irons, blow dryers and other appliances to help with our hair. Whether short, long, orange, blond, even purple, ten-year-olds can choose how they want to wear their hair. Braids are a luxury. Today, I keep a natural short, brushed look.

We had family time with Bible readings every night. Sometimes we sang hymns, and one of my favorites was, "On Christ The Solid Rock I Stand." I still love how it reminds me to never lose the power God gave me. I didn't know what it meant as a child, but I definitely know now.

# DADDY'S 7-UP REQUIREMENTS

1. Wake up at 7:00 a.m.

2. Get up quickly, no last minute snoozes.

3. Get ready in 30 minutes. Say your prayers, wash up, brush your teeth, and get into the kitchen.

4. Get to breakfast on time or there would be none left for you.

5. Shut up the fuss with your siblings. Don't chat too much.

6. Report for duty in a timely manner.

7. Don't go too slow in the field or you would hear Daddy say, "Speed up!"

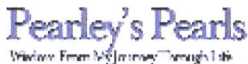

Pearley's Pearls
Wisdom From My Journey Through Life

## Heartfelt Prayers As a Child

One of the lessons I carry with me is about the importance of prayer. We prayed as a family, and it was something that meant a lot to us all. When prayer was disbanded in school, Mother told us to pray in our hearts. As a child I didn't know what it meant to pray in my heart. *"How can I pray without speaking?"* I asked myself. I didn't understand it all then, but when Hurricane Hazel hit the schools, I started praying.

My siblings and I attended a two-room school called Concord Elementary, it had a potbelly stove in the middle of the floor. That was the only school in our area, and we attended there until I was in the fifth grade. The Principal, Rev. McFadden, and his wife, Mrs. McFadden, taught us the "Good Morning" song that we sang every morning. When schools were integrated, I wasn't excited that we had to be bussed to B.F. Person School in Franklinton, North Carolina.

It was a fall day in 1954, when Hurricane Hazel came to Franklin County. Rev. McFadden didn't close school early for us to make it home in time to shelter in from the bad storm. It was October 15th, and all of us were running home in strong winds blowing 110 miles per hour. Lethal debris was flying over our heads. We were ducking and dodging dog house tops, tree limbs, buckets, chairs, brooms, and the list goes on. It was the Grace of God that gripped our feet to the ground until we made it home. That storm claimed many lives and even today, it's still chilling to talk about it.

I don't know how it ended up just being my classmate, Johnnie, and me running together. We clenched hands tightly and held on for dear life, as we ran. I never held another boy's hand before that day, except my brothers.

Bob Harrison was our only means of new information. He was on the 5:00 p.m. news every day. Mother said that day he had come across the air frequently saying that everyone should stay off of the road. Daddy stayed home, not realizing that we were going to get caught in the storm.

Mother was standing at the door with open arms waiting for us. She told Johnnie that his grandparents were worried about him. He wanted to keep running further down the road to his house, but Mother thought it was best if he remained with us until the storm ceased.

Our greatest loss from the storm was that our mules, our prime vehicles on the farm, were struck by lightning. We didn't have cars like people do today. Many homes and businesses were also struck by lightning. Daddy was saying, "I don't know what I'm going to do," over and over. He was so upset.

What a friend we have in Jesus! God works in mysterious ways. My brothers were elevated from walking behind the mules (Woo-hoo), to a riding tractor to do their chores. Let the praise time begin!

I learned from this catastrophe that in the storms of life we may be tossed and turned, but we need to pick up the debris and move on.

I can still remember where I was standing in the MAC Gymnasium when Mr. Keck spoke over the intercom in a panic, "President John F. Kennedy has been assassinated." It felt like time stopped. I looked around and the students were frozen in place. It was shocking and hurtful news for everyone, especially in our small Black community. I prayed in my heart that day. None of us knew what was next, but we believed that God would come through.

I was standing on God's Word that He is our refuge and a very present help in the time of trouble as it is written in Psalm 46:1.

## High School

I played on the junior varsity basketball team for two years. Mother was the oldest of six girls, and it was a generational belief that girls should be home at night. Mother told me a story about how she got in trouble one time because one of her sisters went across the road being nosy, and Mother was punished because she was watching her.

She was so strict that, when my high school basketball team traveled to different schools to play games, I couldn't go. Mother only allowed me to play at night when we had a home game at school. Bertha and Virginia were my best friends, and they knew how strict Mother was. Daddy convinced Mother to let me play, and he would take me to the games. I had to be in the door at 9:00 p.m., not 9:01 p.m..

When I went to the prom, Mother even made my brother, Alphonso come home from New Jersey to take me. He brought his fiancée with him, and she stayed at the house.

Back in the day having a phone was a luxury. We used the Vance County telephone exchange; sometimes, as many as four families shared the same line. Mother and Daddy agreed we could have a phone, but they gave us conditions. We all knew that we weren't supposed to make long distance calls; the phone was for emergencies only. Our parents did allow us to talk to a friend for a few minutes on Saturdays, if we had all of our chores done.

Our monthly telephone bill was normally around $9.68. One month when the bill came, it was $11.38 and Daddy put Mother on the case to find out why the bill was so high. It took her about a month to complete her investigation. After she interrogated all of us and determined the cause, Mother reported to Daddy that there were two calls made to New Jersey. Everyone turned their eyes to me, because I had been sneaking on the line calling my boyfriend.

Daddy shut it down quickly, bam! No phone for any of us. There was not one chance to say, "I won't do it again." My siblings still tease me about those phone calls. I truly didn't think anyone would find out. The moral to this story is: be mindful when you disobey because you will face consequences. No matter how small, you not only hurt yourself when you disobey, but you can also hurt others.

Life is all about the lessons we learn.

*A time to be born, a time to die,*
*a time to plant and a time to pluck up*
*what's planted.*
*A time to kill, a time to heal,*
*a time to breakdown*
*a time to build up.*
*A time to be mourn a time laugh,*
*a time to dance.*

Ecclesiastes 3:2-4

*"To everything there is a season, and a time to every purpose under the heaven."*

Ecclesiastes 3:1 (KJV)

# TO EVERYTHING THERE IS A SEASON

New days bring transformation to our souls. Even though seasons change, we have to find the strength to rise every day with hope and faith.

## Spring

As a child, Spring was considered the sweetest season for me because it represented new beginnings. Three times weekly, we had to pluck cucumbers early in the morning while dew was still dripping from the vine. I hated getting up early for that chore.

One day I was tired of picking them thangs, and I fed some to the cow, but Daddy saw me. He was preparing for his truck farming sales season and giving those cucumbers to the cow was taking away from our family's income. I never thought he would spank me, but I paid dearly because Daddy did have to spank me. It hurt him so much, because he had never spanked me before, I was the oldest girl.

Daddy cried after he disciplined me; that was my second time ever seeing him cry, but his tears remained our secret until around 2014.

The first time I saw Daddy cry was when his brother, Uncle William, and other family members perished in a train accident. When Daddy got the news, he stood by the fireplace and sobbed. Mother said we were too small to go to the funeral.

## Summer

Summer vacation from school meant down home traditions for our family. We didn't need an alarm clock because Daddy was an early riser, and he utilized his "7-UP" agenda during that time of the year. He let us sleep in a little later, but our chores did not change. Two of my chores were to feed the chickens and restock the bird feeder. Mother used to kiss at the red cardinals, whenever she saw them.

The boys tended to the pigs and milked the cows. We had to do our laundry, and most of the time we made soap powder from the oils of the pigs. We each had to iron our sheets, dress our beds, and iron our clothes.

My sister, Carolyn, and I had to wash dishes every other night. I don't know how, but one night we broke all of the plates. We got a whipping from Mother, and I still remember her telling Daddy. They had to get new plates for us.

After we had done our chores, Daddy would find a watermelon behind a cool vine. He would carry it up to the house, burst it open on the cement porch, and we would eat it up!

## Fall

In the Fall we prepared for the sale of tobacco and cotton. Everyone was on their best behavior because it was harvest time. We would sell our goods to cover our livelihood. Daddy was usually easygoing and cool, but during this season, he was more like a drill sergeant. If Daddy wasn't happy . . . nobody was happy.

On a dark autumn evening in 1957, we experienced our worst nightmare; back then we worked at different locations to harvest land. That night, we were a mile from home working on a different location to harvest tobacco for sale. We heard loud screaming, and Grover Lee, one of our neighbors, started beating on the door. He was shouting, "Mr. Joe and Mrs. Sallie Lou, your house is on fire."

Daddy opened the door and said, "NO!"

Grover Lee said, "Look!" We could see the fire, we jumped into the truck, and Daddy drove it as fast as it would go.

When we saw our house we couldn't believe it. The roof was falling in, while bright orange and red sparks along with black smoke billowed from our home.

Daddy tried to go inside and the neighbors were shouting, "Come back! Come back! Don't go in there!"

I can still feel Mother and Daddy holding us tight saying, "Everything will be alright." After the fire, all we had were the clothes on our backs and the clothes hanging on the line.

I wanted my doll and tea set. Carolyn wanted her private notebook. My oldest brother, Alfonza, wanted his tool box. Until the day she died from gall bladder cancer, I don't think Mother ever stopped looking for our baby pictures. I remember her looking in drawers, her hat closet, and the cedar chest at the foot of her bed trying to recapture the memories of us.

There was no social media back then, but news spread fast about our loss. At that time, I had not heard of the "Serenity Prayer," used by many support groups. It was written by Dr. Reinhold Niebuhr, of the Union Theological Seminary, in 1932. There is a line in his poem that is very popular, "God grant me the serenity to accept the things I cannot change; courage to change the things I can; and wisdom to know the difference." As a family, we had no choice but to except the things we couldn't change.

Cousins Laura and Isaiah Sneed opened their hearts and home after hearing my brother ask, "Where are we going to sleep?" Cousin Laura invited him to stay with them, because she was glad to have a companion for her son, Richard. She welcomed him into her home because they had all girls and one boy in their house. He was with them for about two weeks. Cousin Laura could sew, and she made us some clothes. Mr. Adolphus and Mrs. Flora Kearney opened their home to us.

The next morning after the fire, Mrs. Flora made golden-brown biscuits and pear preserves for us. We savored the food then rushed down the hill to our house where Daddy and a neighbor had stood all night. Seeing my Daddy reach into the debris and ashes with his bare hands to see what he could salvage reminded me of why Grandma called him, "Gold." I think he was hoping to find something to help us move forward. In that moment with his hands in the ashes, I saw how Grandma's vision about him proved to be true.

## Rebuilding

Daddy was creative. Before the fire, he was in the process of expanding the barn for our mules. After the fire, he immediately began rebuilding the barn. Daddy applied some of the skills he learned working in the community, and his handiwork resulted in him redesigning our house.

Our neighbors helped Daddy rebuild, and he called it our "Holding Place." He added two large rooms and a kitchen with a room divider for him and Mother's privacy. The neighbors helped him build the barn in seven days, so we would have some place to stay and not be separated.

When we moved into the barn the fresh aroma of hay tickled my nose. I thought about Jesus when He was born in a manger. We could see our livestock through gaps in the walls that weren't tightly sealed.

We could hear Daddy and Mother whispering through the walls saying that the contractors had missed closing dates. The insurance company took a long time to settle, but when they did, we had a brand new brick house built from the ground.

Through faith, our family was able to come together. We were supported by the community who rallied around us and supported us during that season of our lives. In addition, donations from churches and individuals were very helpful and meant more than words could express. We were able to visit a local mission organization for other resources. The owner of the mission reminded us that we needed to wash everything before we used it.

I am grateful God spared my family and provided resources in our time of need. This is why as an adult, I am intentional about helping other people. One Sunday at UBC, my pastor invited the director of a Rescue Mission to speak to the congregation. He told a story about how when he was a child, his house had burned down. He started the mission to help other families. I knew when he mentioned that story, that my family had been blessed by a rescue and a mission, when we were able to get resources.

## Winter

Even though the fire happened in the fall of the year, it represented a winter season for my family spiritually, emotionally and mentally. Usually in the winter, all life seems to cease and that's what happened for us. Our house had been destroyed. We were looking for our memories. Our family had been separated. In that season, I felt cold, and losing everything felt like the leaves were falling off of me.

Thankfully, that December, we were gifted a Christmas tree, and we were overjoyed about Santa coming down the chimney with our toys and gifts as usual. All praises to God, we had a great Christmas dinner. Daddy purchased a hot plate with three cooking eyes. We cooked fried chicken, apple jacks and collard greens at a little slower pace, yet it didn't change the taste of the food.

As the year went on, we had visits from the Easter Bunny and the Tooth Fairy, too. I believe that Daddy and Mother didn't build a mega house; they didn't have a Cadillac in the garage, or a 401K in the bank. We had love, and that kept us together.

The winter season was difficult, but we got through it. I gathered some pearls of wisdom which are valuable to me because, I believe that when I survived the winter season, God gave me true wealth. Even though we lost our house, we gained so much more. God strengthened my faith, and I recognized that wealth is more than money and material things.

As an adult, I learned that true wealth is not measured by material things, but by the treasures or the pearls of wisdom that God provides. Here is a pearl of wisdom for you: go deep inside of your heart to obtain true spiritual wealth. That is where only your spirit and God dwells.

## Our New Home

Daddy and Mother were strong vessels. Despite the tragedy, as a family, we were survivors. When we rose in our new brick home on Easter Sunday morning, our souls were magnified. Mother stood in the house with her Bible open to Isaiah 40:31 and read: "But they that wait upon the LORD shall renew *their* strength; they shall mount up with wings as eagles; they shall run, and not be weary; *and* they shall walk, and not faint." I still get emotional thinking about it.

Every time I hear of someone losing their home to fire, the tape begins rolling of our prior tragedy. We will never get the photos, our favorite doll, tea set, toolbox, or notebook, but we did get our strength renewed. During this struggle, I heard Mother and Daddy say numerous times that our whole life's earnings were gone. What we thought was our worst nightmare turned into a touch of glory from God, because He restored everything.

Every time I hear the Christmas story, I picture my family sleeping with the livestock like Jesus born in the manger wrapped in swaddling clothes, and my praises go up. When I hear the Easter story, I hear John the Baptist shouting, "Behold the Lamb of God who takes away the sins of the world." Then I hear the Angel saying, "He's is not there, for He is risen."

As I have grown into adulthood, I have learned that there are no guarantees in life. It can take a lifetime to build and mold a castle, and with one strong wind or spark, everything can come tumbling down in a matter of minutes.

## "Gold"

My daddy passed on December 30, 1989. At his funeral on January 3, 1990, we heard wonderful stories about him from our family. After his father died, he was chosen by Grandma to go work in the community while his brothers stayed and worked on the farm. Daddy worked and learned skilled trades from other cultures and brought what he learned back home. It was a surprise to all of us to hear our Uncle Dave say, "Mama always called Brother Joe, 'Gold,' because everything he touched turned to gold."

I often think about the lessons my parents taught me, and when the image of Daddy standing at the fireplace grieving comes to mind, I realize that in my young mind, I wondered if Daddy was ever going to be himself again. When I learned that Grandma called him "Gold," it gave me the true question I was pondering that day as a child, "Will my Daddy ever be gold again?" I couldn't comprehend the weight of what he was carrying. I now have the pearls of wisdom from Proverbs 17:3

*In the same way that gold and silver are refined by fire, the Lord purifies your heart by the tests and trials of life.* (The Passion Translation)

My parents had hearts of pure gold, and I thank God for them.

*"I will never leave you
or forsake you."*

~Hebrews 13:5

# FOOTPRINTS IN THE SAND

Footprints in the sand is what it was like for us at the beach. Our prints in the sand and the written word on our hand. Our hearts crying, "Hallelujah" with psalms of praise.

I've been revived. I've been revived.

Then we assembled inside and united in name to worship Christ our Lord. We forgot about ourselves and everyone else.

Then the buffet was spread. We all had the same entree; we were fed so much we wanted to stay. From a menu of gifts of discovery, joy, godliness, and fitness.

When we thought we had all that one could eat, we were served with dessert - a jump start of stagnant spiritual life. No wonder we were more physically fit and ready for the action plan and the job possibilities.

Now we all have taken a new route from our footprints in the sand to sowing into our birthright talents and being more gifted, Godly and growing in the field where we have been transformed.

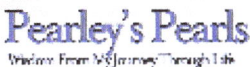

Pearley's Pearls
Wisdom From My Journey Through Life

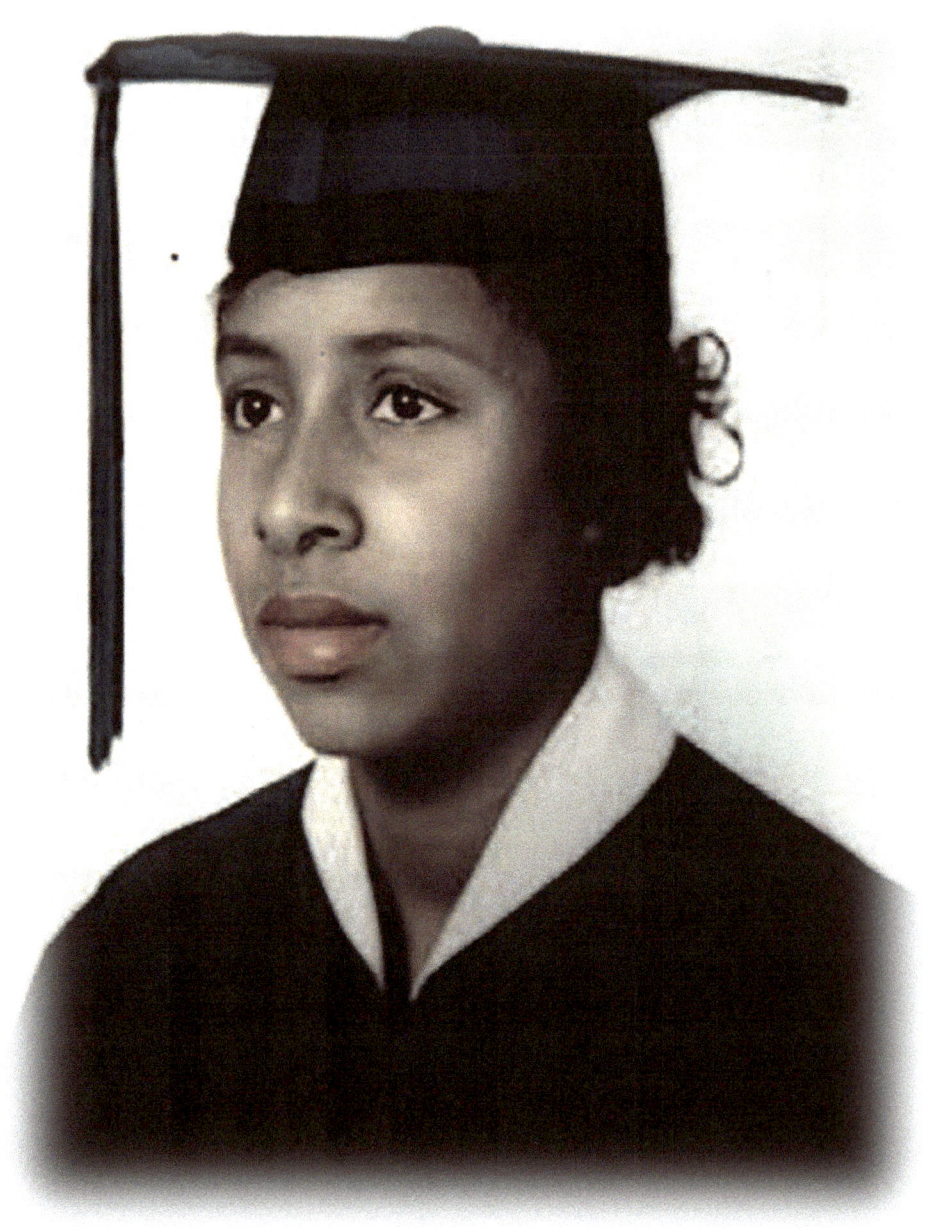

# LEAVING HOME

I graduated from B.F. Person High School in Franklinton, North Carolina in May of 1964. Mother and Daddy weren't happy that I decided to leave home to attend W.W. Holden Technical College in Raleigh, North Carolina. They told me that it was my decision, and I left for college in August.

Daddy's health was declining, and he wasn't doing well with his arthritis and mild case of tuberculosis. For a while, he couldn't work at all, he would only find comfort in his rest. To keep the farm going, Mother and Daddy had to hire help. I know that he wanted me to stay and help, but he also wanted me to get a higher education.

I didn't have anything in mind that I really wanted to study in college. I knew that I always wanted to work in the hospital, but no particular field came to mind. I just knew that I had to go.

The day that I left home, my family took me to the Trailways bus station. It was a sad time; we cried and hugged each other before I got on the bus. I was worried about my little sister who was still at home. Beverly is twelve years younger, and she asked me, "Pearley, who is going to comb my hair?"

My parents said in their own words, "I taught you how to be a lady, and now you have to step out and be a woman." As the bus pulled off, I knew I was leaving the nest to pursue my own dreams. I had to trust God to bless my version of faith.

## Ms. Shaw's Boarding House

My high school teacher and senior advisor, Ms. Dorothy Jones, lived in Raleigh. She had recommended a boarding house where I could live that was not too far from the school. When I arrived in Raleigh at the bus station, I hailed a taxi to take me to Ms. Shaw's house.

When I took my suitcase out of the car I felt strange. Ms. Shaw greeted me and said, "Come on in, honey." She gave me a tour of the house and took me to my bedroom. She had three bedrooms, and there were three other young ladies around my age already there. I was the youngest of the group. I became close with my housemates, and they were like a second family.

We all shared a kitchen, a bathroom, and a sitting room. I was using money that I had saved to pay my rent, which was only ten dollars a week. I stepped out on nothing and landed on something that was carved out for me. God showed me the mustard seed faith I had heard about all of my life. By the third week, I realized that my money was running out. In my parents' house, the bacon was free. When I had to put the bacon on my own table, I realized that my upbringing had given me a strong desperation for my destiny.

My roommate, Catherine, mentioned that there was an opening at the restaurant where she was a waitress. I got a job washing dishes, but after about a week and a half, I resigned from that job. Washing dishes was not for me!

After leaving my job, I realized that the tobacco roads I came from weren't so bad after all. My upbringing taught me how not to give up, it gave me tenacity and strengthened my perseverance. I started thinking about who I was when I was back home. I was the secretary for my Junior Sunday School class. I wrote poems, I read the finance reports in front of church, and I used to be in charge of Children's Day. I recognized that I didn't want to be back home, but I needed to do something different and find myself. I had to find where God wanted me.

At night when I would go back to my room, I would think about all the things I wanted to be. I was always an ambassador, and I was born and reared to write, discover, and produce. It did not take long for me to learn that where I came from didn't define me, it shaped me. Through all of this reflection, I can see how God was pulling on my heart and taking me in the direction of my destiny.

*"Clarence and I lived all of our vows: for richer or poorer, in sickness and in health."*

~Pearley Long Yelverton

# MEETING MY BOO

About a week after I quit my job, Catherine suggested that we ditch class. "Come on, let's skip class," she said with a smile. "I want to go out with my boyfriend."

I said to her, "What do you mean skip school? I never heard anything about that." I knew that wasn't why Mother sent me to school. At first, I felt like I was letting Mother down, but after some consideration, I decided to go with her.

When Catherine's boyfriend arrived, to pick us up from the school, he had one of his buddies in the car. Clarence got out of the front seat and got into the back. Catherine's boyfriend introduced me to Clarence, as she got in the front seat.

We went to a restaurant and ate hamburgers. I was used to hotdogs, "wieners," as we called them, so eating burgers was a new experience for me. That day Clarence and I ended up talking for a long while. We discussed his family, my family, and his job as an orderly in the hospital. I remember the way that he looked at me, it was different.

After about four hours of talking, Clarence said, "You are going to be my wife."

I thought he was just talking, but what he was saying made me feel safe. There was something about him. I knew that I didn't want to wash any more dishes, and when he told me that we could have a home together, I believed him. He had already prepared a home for himself and his mother. It was a lot to take in at that time, but there was something different about Clarence.

In high school, I had dated a minister. We grew up together in church, but when he went off to college, he met another girl and started dating her. They ended up getting married in our church. I was so hurt from that experience, but when I was with Clarence, I felt that he was the person for me. He used to sing the song by Roberta Flack and Donny Hathaway, "The First Time Ever I Saw Your Face," because it represented our love story.

## A Proposal

After dating Clarence for three months, I said, "I'd like for you to meet my parents."

"Sure," he said, "I was wondering when you were going to ask." I wrote to Mother and asked if I could bring him home. She wrote me back and told me it was okay. Two weeks later, when Clarence's schedule was solidified, his coworker drove us in his Studebaker to Kittrell, NC. Clarence could drive, but he did not want to drive the forty-five mile distance. At the time, he was experiencing the onset of his hereditary vision problem.

When we pulled up, Mother and Daddy were waiting for us. It was kind of scary in the beginning, but I could tell after a while they really liked each other.

Daddy talked to Clarence. Mother talked to Clarence. Then Mother and Daddy talked to Clarence. They were impressed with him, because he had taken care of his mother after his parents separated. They knew that if a man could take care of his mother, he would take care of his wife.

After five hours of their "interrogation," as he called it, Clarence asked me to marry him again. He had purchased a ring, and I realized he had planned it all out, but it was a surprise to me.

"He is out of his mind," I thought, but I said, "Yes." Ironically, the first time I skipped class, I met my Boo, and started a new life.

## The Wedding Day

We chose the date February 22, 1965, to exchange our vows. The pastor's schedule was open on that Monday, yet we did not realize it was a holiday. Once we learned that it was, we chose to sneak out and take advantage of the sales. Clarence and I slipped away early that morning, even though we knew the superstition said he was not supposed to see me before the wedding. It was so much fun purchasing items for our home at the twenty-two cents sale. Thankfully, God broke all of those old wives' tales off of us.

I happily exchanged my schooling for the gift of marriage and family responsibilities. Clarence had been a playboy before we got together, his mother knew when she met me that I was the one for him.

We were young and optimistic, when we had our candlelight evening wedding. in the home he shared with his mother. Clarence's brother-in-law, Robert King, was the best man, and Robert's wife, Geraldine was the witness. My beautiful Mother-In-Law, Beatrice A. Yelverton, used to hum, "Amazing Grace" around the house. She lit the candles for us, but didn't stay in the room for the ceremony.

## Here Come The Children

Our first-born, Clarence Yelverton, Jr., tipped the scales at 2.2 pounds, when he was born in 1966 the next year. Our baby was premature because I had preeclampsia. I had a seizure when I gave birth, because my blood pressure was up. We could only see our baby through the NICU walls. He passed away on Mother's Day. I guess God knew that my baby needed more intense love and care.

Our son, Grear, was born healthy September 10, 1967; however, Bernard was born premature on November 8, 1968, at 2.11 ounces. That brought back some of the grief I had experienced with our first son, Clarence, Jr. By God's grace, Bernard survived, and our daughter, Nikki, came seven years later on March 24, 1975. We didn't know she was coming, but she was a wonderful surprise for us all.

Every Sunday afternoon, I would watch my Clarence sit on the floor with our children. Whenever he would say, "A song is not a song until you sing it," I was reminded of my Grandpa. When I was a child, my Grandpa gave my brother a ball. I was always fascinated by the ball. One day I got a chance to roll and rub it. When Grandpa saw me playing with it, he said, "Baby, let me show you how it works. A ball is not a ball until you bounce it."

Despite seeing each other, God smiled on the forty-eight years He gave us in marriage. We bloomed with fruit and were blessed throughout our days. Clarence and I lived all of our vows: for richer or poorer, in sickness and in health until death separated us on June 19, 2014.

*"Sometimes life takes you all the way down, in order to bring you back up, even better than before."*

~Pearley Long Yelverton

# CHANGING DIRECTIONS

Clarence and I had good times when we were first married and young. He worked a second shift job from 3:00 p.m. to 11:00 p.m. at Wilson Memorial Hospital. When he would get off of work and arrived at home, he would put his key in the door and call out for me, "Pudding. Pudding, I'm home."

I would be waiting up for him. At that time, I didn't know anybody in Wilson other than him and my mother-in-law. Mother Yelverton was so kind to me. Most days she would either be asleep or worshiping in her apostolic church.

In 1967, Clarence's vision began to deteriorate. At a doctor's appointment, the physician told him that he needed to change jobs. As it turns out, Clarence couldn't see the thermometer that well to take the temperature of his patients. The doctor recommended that he enroll in the School for the Blind and Deaf in Garner, North Carolina. Clarence's brother, Gene, and his wife, Louise Yelverton lived in Durham. Garner is around forty-five miles from Durham, so it was not going to be a bad commute for Clarence to get to school.

I was so happy when we moved to Durham. Living in "The Bull City," had always been my dream. I heard that Durham had great homes, a strong family living environment, enormous employment opportunities, outstanding healthcare, good schools, and several universities. Most importantly, Durham is a city of great faith for praise and worship.

I was grateful that Clarence could expand his skill set at the School for the Blind. While he was in training, he was given an opportunity to work at the Lion's Club for the blind. There had never been an African American in management at the Lion's Club; Clarence was the first. He was good at his job, and they transported him to school and work.

Life was good in Durham those first few years. Clarence loved his job. He did experience some pressure in his new role, but he had so much joy. The job gave us many new opportunities such as: the ability to buy a house, cars, and other material things that we probably didn't need.

## Working at Union Baptist Church

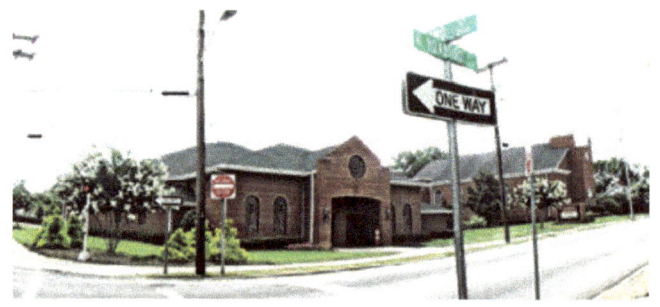

My first job in Durham was at Union Baptist Church (UBC); I worked in Head Start. I am proud to say that UBC was the first church in Durham that accepted that program. Our son, Grear was in Head Start, and I would often go check on him in his classroom. One day I went in his class and the director said, "Mrs. Yelverton, why don't you come and volunteer with us?"

After a few times volunteering, I was offered a job with Grear's classroom. Even though Clarence wanted me to stay home with the children, I loved working with the three and four year olds. The job brought back fond memories of when I volunteered with my 4-H club back home. I used the tools I learned from that time in my classroom.

Clarence and I both had jobs we loved. God had given us the "American Dream" of love, marriage, and children. I met my good friend, Alois while working at UBC. She introduced me to her husband, Micheal, and their children. Our families grew close over the years.

My coworkers frequently talked about the Executive Director who was a man with a mighty big name in the community. They were afraid of him, because they perceived him as being a man with a bad attitude. If they saw him coming down the hall at work, they would cross to the other side to avoid him. Their worries about him didn't bother me much. I didn't see what they saw. Even though I wasn't into, "the Jesus stuff," back then, I knew Jesus was a man with all power. I guess all of those boring breakfast prayers Mother prayed before we could eat, had strengthened my faith and kept me protected and sustained since childhood.

## No Longer Needed

After being at UBC for a few months, I arrived to work one morning and was informed by my supervisor, "After 5:00 you will no longer be needed." They gave me no explanation for why I was being let go. I was confused, because I had been given a good evaluation the week before. That morning, I was happy when I arrived at work, but the news that I was being let go took the air out of my spiritual tires.

People have told me all of my life that I needed to speak up for myself. I wish I had utilized the skill of self-advocacy the day I was let go. Instead, I left my job at the church feeling how Humpy Dumpty must have felt when he fell off of the wall. Believe me, I felt the devastation of that fall. At the time, none of the Kings or Queens could have put me back together again, just like Humpty Dumpty.

I called the Executive Director's office that Monday morning and scheduled an appointment for 3:00. Upon arrival to his office on East Main Street, I was greeted by his sweet secretary. I had never seen her before, yet she welcomed me warmly. I was appreciative of her and thanked her for her kindness before she led me into Mr. Executive Director's office.

When I saw him, I thought about what Mother often said, "If you open your mouth, God will speak for you with professionalism and compassion."

Entering his office, I began with cordial greetings, and I said, "Thank you for seeing me on such a short notice." Mr. Executive Director offered me a seat in front of his desk. I shared with him the news that I was fired. The look of shock on his face let me know that he wasn't aware I had been let go from my job.

Mr. Executive Director said, "You should know that there are a lot of changes in federal funding." I was listening to what he said, and his bottom line was, "Last hired, first fired."

He called his secretary and asked her to bring a job list. She brought some documents into the office, and he looked them over. "Ah," he said, "we have one position that needs to be filled immediately. It's a Mail Clerk position."

"I will take it, sir."

He looked pleasantly surprised. "It will be about two weeks before the position is ready for you." Even though women didn't shake hands, I stood and shook his hand with excitement.

"I loved those cute little four and five year-olds at the daycare," I thought. "But, God has elevated me." Little did I know that the elevation was to my own office; with my name on the door!

In the mail room there was a lot of Pitney Bowes equipment to help me do my job effectively. My supervisor was a cool lady who knew about the equipment and taught me what I needed to know. "Pearley," she said, "sometimes you have to fake it until you make it." I did that, until I got comfortable with all of the machines.

My new job came with medical insurance, retirement benefits and a big salary increase. I was so excited when the company purchased a brand new yellow Pinto from the dealer showroom for me. I used that car to pick up my boys from school and transport my husband to and from work. I had the privilege of taking a break during the day to take care of my family and go back to complete my work assignments. My new job was truly a gift.

One pearl of wisdom that I learned from that job was that sometimes life takes you all the way down in order to bring you back up, even better than before. I am a living witness that when a door closes, a window swings open at the right place and the right time.

Let the praise time begin!

# BAD NEWS

I was diagnosed with breast cancer in July of 1976, when I was twenty-nine. I was touched by cancer, but, from the moment it was diagnosed, I believed that I was a survivor and an overcomer, because of my resilience. It was beyond our wildest nightmare that I had breast cancer.

Hearing the word, "cancer," the first thing I thought about was that I was dying. I prayed constantly, "Please let me see my babies get grown." All praises to God, I was blessed to see them graduate from college with multiple degrees.

We were into the second day of vacation enjoying each other, when we decided to visit Clarence's mother in Wilson, North Carolina. Driving to my Mother-in-Law's home, I experienced an intense pain in my stomach and had to pull over. After a few minutes, when the pain did not subside, Clarence directed me, "Drive directly to the Emergency Room."

## Mittelschmerz

I drove to Wilson Memorial Hospital where Clarence had worked for seventeen years. I ended up being hospitalized for three-days, because they could not find out what was wrong with me. I kept asking what was wrong, and no one mentioned that they had found a lump in my breast.

What they did say was I had "Mittelschmerz," which is mostly seen in European women. I had never heard anything about it. It surprised the doctors that I was a colored woman with symptoms. Clarence and I knew that we were facing something serious, because the doctors were interviewing many females from Mother's family for their medical history.

Mittelschmerz is pain between a menstrual cycle when the egg is released from the ovary. They treated me with strong medication to alleviate the pain. Three days later, when I was finally released from the hospital, I could not drive. A family member came and drove us back to Durham to take me to the "Colored Hospital," Lincoln Memorial.

After being at Lincoln for three days, the doctors realized that Wilson Memorial had authorized a direct admission to Duke University Medical Center, "the big hospital." Lincoln Memorial also chose not to mention that there was a lump in my breast. I had three admissions within nine days from that belly ache. I was confused and didn't know what to expect when I went to Duke Medical Center.

We had to call on our families to pick up the children because things were erratic.

## Breast Cancer?

On Sunday, August 15, my room was surrounded with family and friends. Clarence was the lead singer for the Sensational Angels, a gospel singing group, and they had a performance out of town that day. As I watched the clock drawing closer to the time he was supposed to leave, I told him, "The group is waiting for you. You can go ahead." Reluctantly, he left.

The doctors who had made an appointment to come and talk to my family burst into the room late after Clarence left. They displayed no compassion or respect for me. The attending interrupted us talking and blurted out, "Mrs. Yelverton the lump in your breast is cancer carcinoma. Your surgery is scheduled for 7:00 tomorrow morning. By the way, NPO after 12:00."

"What lump is he talking about?" I wondered. "What is NPO? Whatever happened to Mittelschmerz?"

My younger sister, Carolyn, my mother, some wives from Clarence's singing group, and Alois were with me in the room. Carolyn stood in her sister role and scolded the doctor, "You never asked if it was okay to discuss this in this room full of her family and friends." They had invaded my privacy; HIPPA wasn't enforced as much back then.

Carolyn was a social worker, and she let him have it. "That should have been between her and her husband, and he is not here right now."

The year I was diagnosed with breast cancer was the year that former President Jimmy Carter was inaugurated into office. I remember it because our daughter, Nikki, was only eighteen months old at the time. I didn't see my baby girl the whole time I was hospitalized and in recovery.

I never forgot what I was taught, "What happens at home stays at home." When Clarence and I caught a moment to breathe we did. We realized that we had been holding so much to ourselves and pushing it under the rug. Trying to keep our burdens to ourselves, we began tripping and falling over everything. We had not been acknowledging some of the hazard signs along the way.

We realized that we had to drop the pride and ask for help. My family came together as my greatest support system. "Mama T," who was our babysitter, was a miracle from heaven. When she found out what was happening, she volunteered to care for my daughter in her home; she brought so much peace for us during that journey.

Mama T was a blessing because my mother lived forty miles away, and my daddy was sick. Sweet Mama T's daughter was a renal nurse, and she traveled to help her mother care for our baby girl. Her compassion relieved some pressure from Clarence who only had the boys to take care of.

### An Intricate Reconstruction

On August 16, 1975, I had a modified radical mastectomy. They removed eighteen lymph nodes from my right arm. I ended up having three surgeries in twenty-one days. After the reconstructive surgery, the nurses followed the doctor's instructions and had my chest banded so tightly, I could barely breathe. After some attempts at loosening it, I literally began removing the bandages. The doctor eventually came and made adjustments for me.

I had a lot of visitors and phone calls. One female coworker called my hospital room and asked, "Pearley, did they really take your titty off?" What do you think, was she ignorant, nosey, or a little bit of both? Another time a family member called and said to me, "Pearley, who would have ever thought, your cousin is gone and you are still here?" Is that cold? Or, is that cold? I didn't even answer her. Mother taught me if I didn't know what to say, to stay silent.

After twenty-one days, I was released from the hospital to go home.

## Chemotherapy

Six weeks after surgery, I started Chemotherapy. The doctors told me I would have eighteen months of oral treatments. It was the same regimen that First Lady Betty Ford did. Chemo changed the texture of my hair, with its mysterious chemicals. I am thankful for my hairstylist, Shirley, at "Shirley's Hairstyles." She began prepping me for the worst by cutting my hair a little each time, and it started growing back. One day she noticed that my hair was changing and suggested, "Why don't you try a short style?" I love my hair short and natural now. I haven't looked back.

## Bad Implants

Doctors informed me that it was possible to have complications from my reconstructive implants. "Give it some time," they said. Unfortunately, I suffered for two months. I had to see a surgeon to follow up on the pain. I had expanders on both arms, and it was so hard for me to keep them in place. I am so glad my caregivers helped me during this time.

It got so painful, I had to return to the doctor. He wasn't available, so, I had to see his son. I didn't sleep that night. I was so afraid of what he might say, but the doctor was very compassionate. He was honest when he said, "The silicone has deflated. It is leaking and corrupting your body." He took a breath and said, "They need to come out right now."

Clarence asked, "Is the damage permanent?"

"Yes," he said lowering his eyes. "They need to come out now. Removing them will take away some of her agony and pain."

Clarence said, "Take them out, enough is enough!" I was back in the hospital within two months, of my original surgery, for yet another surgery to remove my implants. The doctor wanted me to go to the hospital that day, but I took time to make preparations for my children. Mother couldn't come, because Daddy was partially paralyzed. My family was concerned about me and stepped up to help us again. We were learning to let go and accept our help.

Cancer is a big word with a lot of questions floating around it. It invaded my privacy, but it did not steal my joy.

## For Those Healed On The Other Side

It has always concerned me when it was said, someone lost their battle with cancer. One of the hardest moments for me was when my dear mother transitioned. My sister Beverly and I were holding her hands, and even when the nurse pronounced her gone at 9:58 p.m., Mother actually breathed again. It hurt so much to let her go, we all loved her. I feel that Mother and so many others have WON their battles, because they are no longer suffering.

To the Survivors Network in the Triangle, those throughout the Globe, and those resting in peace, we are all survivors and are forever connected.

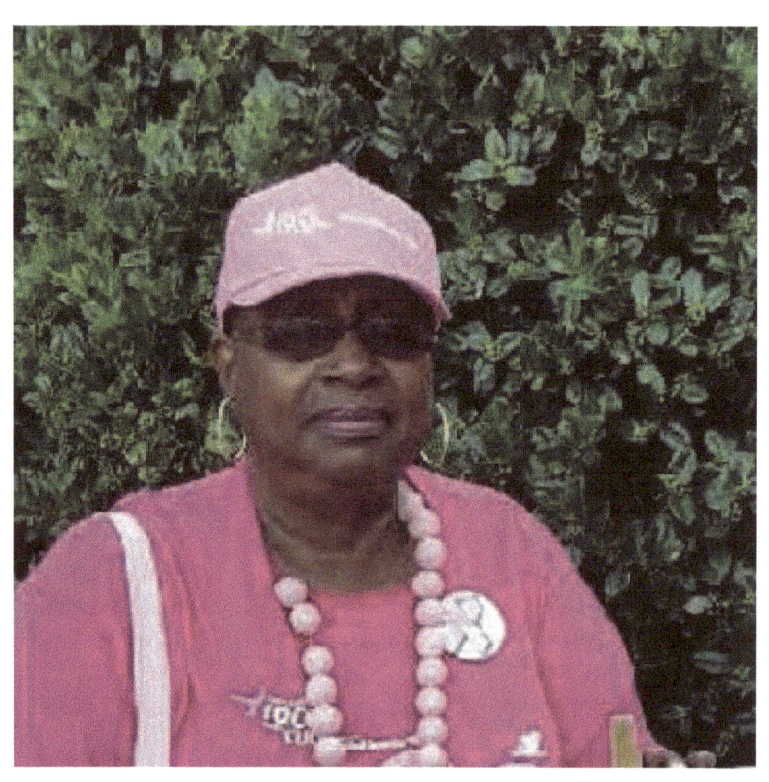

# I AM A SURVIVOR

On New Year's Eve in 2010, fireworks were bursting into flames, horns were blowing, while people were in merriment shaking hands, toasting, and singing, "Auld Lange Syne." It was quite different for Clarence and me. He said I was screaming and hollering because my head was spinning. I was experiencing vertigo, so we went to the hospital. It was sad that we had to miss New Year's Eve worship service.

My head felt like it was on the Ferris wheel at the state fair and Clarence held me in his arms. After a three hour stay in the Emergency Room, I was being prepped for discharge. A doctor and the nursing staff came running in my room saying, "Someone is looking out for you." I didn't know what they were talking about. I wanted to know why I couldn't go home. The doctors said, "You can't go home, we need to admit you into the hospital."

"Why?"

"Mrs. Yelverton, your heart stopped twice." I was diagnosed with Wencke-Bach phenomenon, a heart condition, alongside a severe case of bronchitis. The doctors at Duke Hospital were concerned about my chest pressure, because I had rheumatic fever as a child.

When Grear returned with the car, eight-year-old Jordyn said, "Daddy, the doctors said if Grandma goes home, she could die." The doctors verified that, I experienced two heart blocks, and they needed to monitor me in the hospital.

I celebrate every Women's Heart Awareness Month in February because that experience taught me how to love my heart, so I could continue to do things I love. I was even honored by Two Triangle Sister "Red Dress Reviews."

## Crystals in My Head

After a couple of days in the hospital, they called a specialist who understood vertigo. She looked into my eyes and said, "You are a candidate for resetting the crystal in your head." I had no idea that crystals were in my head. She scheduled me for an outpatient procedure to turn the table upside down and reroute the crystals in my head. I had to sit up for twelve hours, to prevent the crystals from falling.

While the Vertigo Monster was in full assault mode, the Greater One was working for my good. That New Year's Eve, Clarence and I really did have a new beginning. Only the grace of God allowed me to win this one. You would think "enough is enough." Let the praise time begin!

## Seeing the Positive

By far this is my most powerful testimony. I have been a breast cancer survivor for more than forty-nine years. I have been blessed with renewed faith, and God has transformed me. I have been able to live with strength and courage.

My beloved cousin, Linda, introduced me to the Susan G. Komen Walk for the Cure. She and my son Grear, put a group together to fundraise for the walk. They named the group after me, "PEARLEY'S PEARLS." I love the name, and the group is one of my cherished treasures!

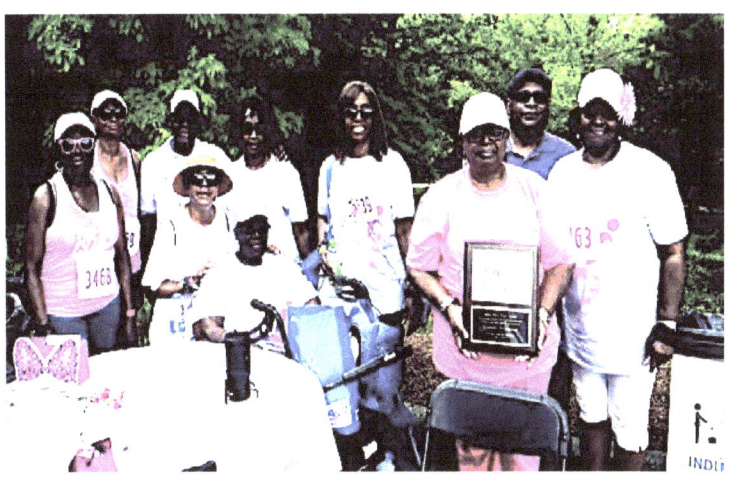

My group has been walking with Susan G. Komen for at least twenty years. I also walked with the American Cancer Society, to raise money and awareness. My first five year survivor photo was with the American Cancer Society, in 1981. I was honored by the Susan G. Komen Triangle Race for the Cure for their "Be Bold. Be Fearless. Be More Than Pink Award," in 2019.

## A Little Soldier

Every year The Susan G. Komen "Breast Cancer Survivor's Walk" is an emotional time for all. My experience in 2012 will always stay with me. I was so excited to be highlighted as one of the longest living survivors in the Triangle area of North Carolina. A group of survivors lined up in a processional and were handed red roses. Two other survivors and I were each assigned a military escort to lead us on stage. There was a special recognition of our cancer being in remission for several years. I was the longest living survivor, and I was feeling a range of emotions.

That particular day, I was last in the procession because I was the longest living survivor. As the last person in line, I was assigned to hold the flag pole to be displayed on stage. The procession was moving slowly and took a long time. As I cradled my rose, feeling tired from standing in line, the escort assigned to me leaned over and said, "I'm so sorry, I'm going to have to leave. I've got another assignment." With that, another escort mentioned that he had to leave also.

I was already crying, because the day was emotional for me thinking about survivors, and those who had received their reward on the other side. When my escort said that he could not stay with me, my tears of joy turned to sadness. "You have to leave?" I asked squeezing my rose.

A ten-year-old child and his family overheard the conversation. I heard a little voice say, "May I carry it for you?" I turned around and thought, *"He is too small to carry the flag pole."* His family looked at me tenderly and warmly said, "Please, let him carry it, he lost his thirty-seven- year-old mother four months ago." That touched my heart. He reached for the tall pole my escort was holding. The flag said, "More than 30 years," it described the number of years I had survived my cancer journey at the time.

The young man escorted me to the stage and made sure I was seated. Before he left the stage, I turned and handed him my rose, which should have gone to a family member. It was a special moment, passing on the rose to him. I wanted to express that I appreciated his support, and that I recognized how losing his mother was a life changing experience. He showed a level of courage and compassion that I couldn't fathom for his age. I will always carry him in my heart.

### Becoming an Advocate

My breast surgeon encouraged me for months to go to Duke Hospital's Administration to complete an application for a job. "They are looking for someone like you to be an ambassador." He said, "I recommended you." When I asked, "Why me?", my surgeon shared that I fit the description of what Duke was looking for in an ambassador. After a few weeks, I received an unexpected call from Human Resources at Duke, and they asked if I would come in and fill out the job application for a Duke Ambassador. I agreed.

I went through three interviews to become the first African American Ambassador of Duke University Medical Center. The job included a salary increase, benefits and college tuition. After careful consideration, I resigned from my mailroom job at Operation Breakthrough to go to Duke Medicine. I was hired for a program called "Reaching For Recovery" with the American Cancer Society. My job was to welcome celebrities and patients when they came to the hospital for their cancer treatments.

God turned my biggest nightmare into one of my greatest accomplishments. I was a little anxious because I was a young, African American woman reaching for recovery myself. I believed that if the Heavenly Father brought me to it, He would take me through it. I was determined to share hope, as I advocated for breast cancer patients. This is my forty-three-year celebration.

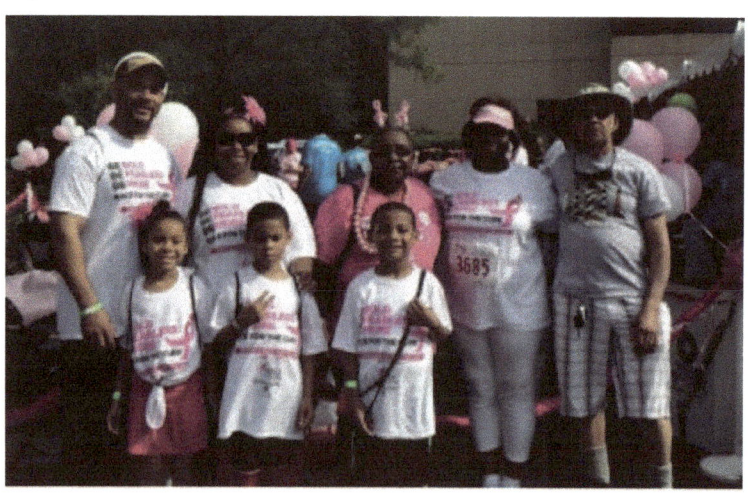

## A Bad Headache

I started working at Duke in 1977. My employer knew I was on chemotherapy when I took the job, and they were receptive. While at work one day, I experienced a bad headache. It was so bad; I regretted all of the times I had ever called out of work, when I didn't really have a headache.

I asked a coworker to switch her fifteen-minute break with me, in hopes to get my headache under control. I sat with my head in my lap, and my hands were shaking. I took so many BC Powders, looking for relief.

I went to the bathroom to get myself together, and I heard a voice say, "Give it to me." I looked around but didn't see anyone. I heard the voice again, "Give it to me." Something beyond human power touched me on my shoulder. Instantly there was no pain, and my body calmed down. I know that it was Jesus who healed me in that bathroom. He met me where I was and healed me. Friend, I have been where you are and have sat where you are sitting. I know what it feels like to sit in the clinic waiting for the lab report to come back.

Now, don't get it twisted, I have known about God my whole life, and I served in church, attended revivals, and sat on the mourner's bench. In my darkest hour, God reassured me of His presence.

I kept my job at the hospital for many years, before becoming disabled because of epilepsy.

1987 EBONETTES SERVICE CLUB
STICK-TO-IT-TIVENESS AWARD
PRESENTED TO
PEARLIE YELVERTON

In 1987, I was awarded the Founder's Day Service Award. Dr. Bernadette Watts shared a heartwarming presentation about me, and I wonder if she remembers how much it touched me. Every time I glimpse at the award on my archive shelf, I am reminded of that Founder's Day Celebration, how it restored me.

"STICK-TO-IT-TIVE-NESS" will never lose its power in me. I remember that whatever God has brought me to, He will bring me through it, because I will stick to it.

# STICK-TO-IT-TIVENESS

After my breast cancer diagnosis, I started seeking new avenues and resources to encourage myself. I loved my job, but I was not happy with myself; breast cancer had changed everything. There were so many processes to help me heal: group psychology, appointments with more doctors, and follow-up appointments with doctors. In the Black culture, seeing a psychologist was not the norm, and I was doing all of those things to help me heal, but I was not feeling fulfilled. No one, in those groups, was my age, and no one looked like me.

I realized that in order for me, as a Black woman to reconstruct and succeed, I needed to surround myself with positive, sharp, astute women to help me rise above setbacks. That's why I responded to a newspaper article that mentioned a women's group called the Ebonettes Service Club. This group was looking for Black women who wanted to impact the lives of others. They served senior citizens, children and young people and I loved their theme, "Lend a helping hand today, see a smiling face tomorrow."

I had to complete an application from the newspaper and submit it to them. A few weeks later, I received a phone call from the membership representative. A formal application was sent to me, and I needed to resubmit it immediately so it was received before the next meeting.

There were a lot of questions on the application and some of them confused me, but I filled it out to the best of my ability. A few days later, I received another call and was invited to the meeting. I was so excited and when I arrived, I was greeted warmly. I admit that I was a little anxious among the well-rounded, articulate self-assured ladies.

Someone from the Membership Department read from my application and introduced me as Pearley Long Yelverton. My application had a lot of blank spaces, and I was totally silent as she read. I could feel the woman's apprehension and I observed her body language as she said, "I don't know what University she attended, what degree she holds, or her status in the Durham, Community." Her words made me feel like a little fish in a very big pond.

One of the Founders, Marjorie L. Thorpe, came over to me and embraced me. She helped me feel better in that moment. While sitting there, the Holy Spirit spoke to me and said, "I have a mission for you in this group and you meet all the requirements. You have your B.A. because you are Born Again."

That day, someone nominated me to be the Chaplain. The motion carried, and I was in office. I never even heard the word Chaplain before. The only term I knew was "Preacher" or "Pastor." I brought nothing into the group, but l left with the duties of Chaplain and a lifetime memory of my dearest friend, Marjorie. Because I was the Chaplain, I was asked to pray at Marjorie's gravesite homegoing services and internment when she passed.

In 2007, I was asked to do the memories and tributes for the Founder's Day Celebration. We honored Marjorie, her beautiful daughter who suddenly passed away from asthma, and Senator Jeanne Hopkins Lucas, the first African American State Senator in North Carolina. I was honored to do their tributes.

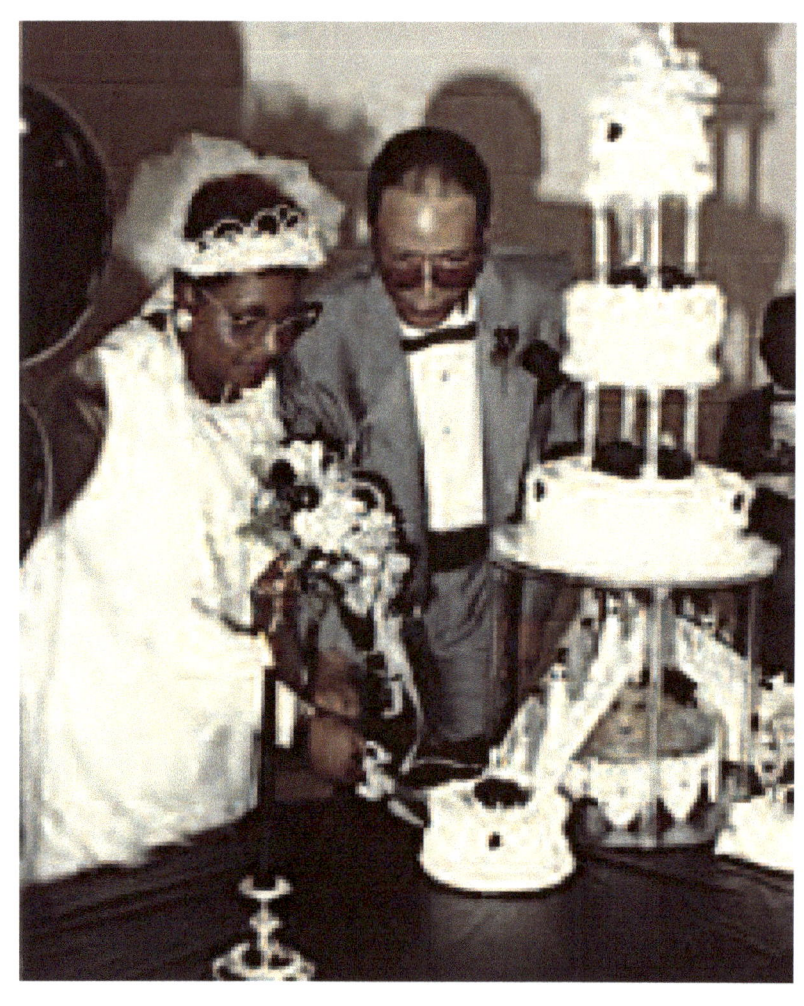

# SILVER WEDDING ANNIVERSARY

On our twenty-fifth wedding anniversary in 1990, Clarence and I renewed our wedding vows. We celebrated with the theme: "God has done great things for us whereof we are glad" (Psalms 126:3). My sister, Dr. Beverly Long Joseph, presided over the ceremony with Pastor Leroy Pegram and his wife, during our vows. Bernard and Nikki sang a song for us, and Grear was able to come home from Air Force duties in Omaha, Nebraska. He was my escort, and it was such a joy to have my children there.

Over the years, Clarence's love, care, wisdom, and strong arms of protection covered me, even when traffic shifted, and I fell into potholes. I always felt safe with him. Celebrating twenty-five years of marriage was monumental for us.

This picture, of Clarence and me with my beloved Aunt Thelma, is so special to me. She came to celebrate with us for our twenty-fifth wedding anniversary, and she was such a pillar in my life. I am so grateful for her because she took care of my family, when I was having seizures. Aunt Thelma was with us over the twelve years I was sick.

This photo, of Clarence and me, is from my sixty-fifth birthday party.

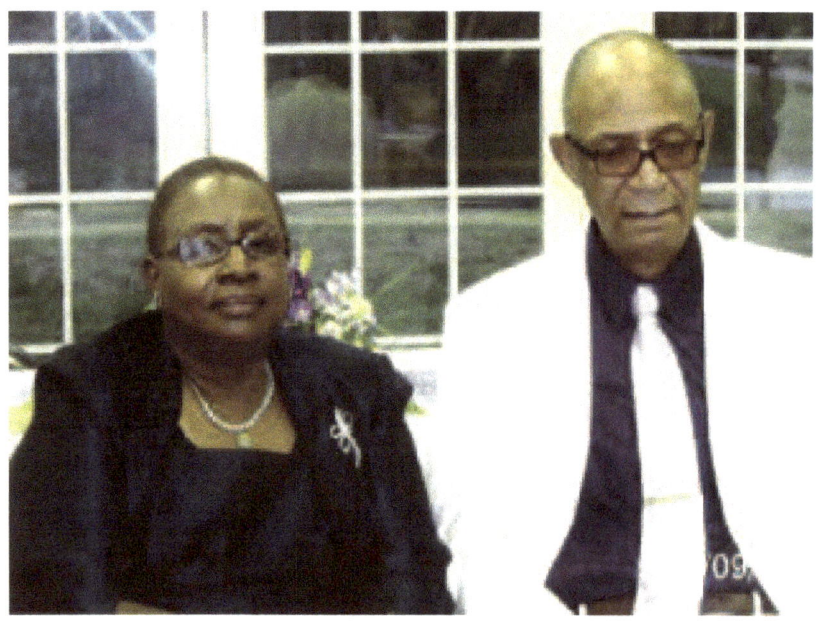

In 2010, we were inducted into the Union Baptist Church "Black Marriage Hall of Fame." This photo is from that day. I was so proud.

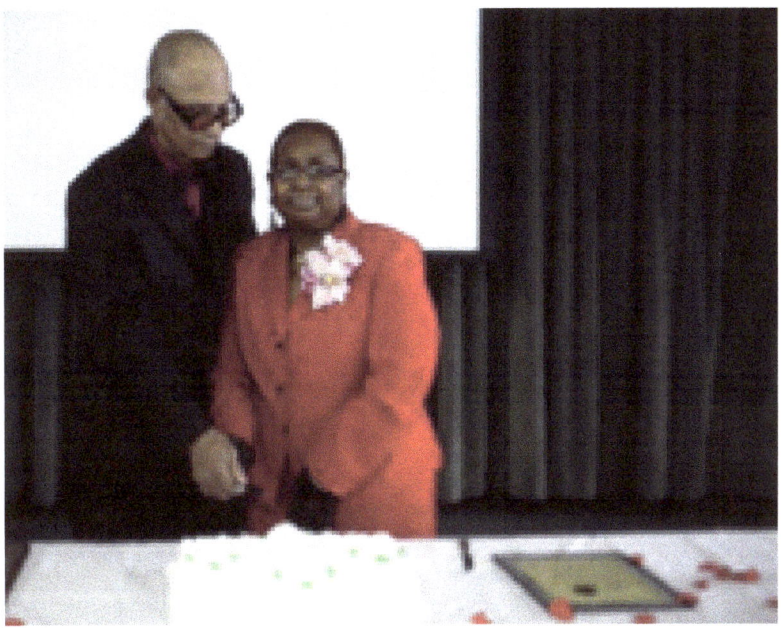

# Union Baptist Church

REVEREND KENNETH RAY HAMMOND
*Senior Minister*

904 N. Roxboro Street • Durham, North Carolina 27701 • (919) 688-1304:1305 • Fax (919) 688-1389
www.unionbaptist-durham.org

March 15, 2010

Dear Mr. and Mrs. Yelverton,

Congratulations!

We are pleased to inform you that you have been selected by the Union Baptist Church Couples Ministry to be inducted into the 2010 Black Marriage Hall of Fame. This event honors those couples who have led by example, holding together their marriages for decades, and whose enduring bond inspires others.

This is UBC's Couples Ministry's third year of joining *Wedded Bliss Foundation* in celebrating the joy of marriage during national Black Marriage Day. The initiative was created by Nisa Muhammad to promote marriage in the Black community in response to bleak statistics about marriage and to create cultural change in the way we look at marriage. Marriage must be celebrated; part of our celebration is in paying tribute to your successful marriage.

The Black Marriage Day Hall of Fame induction will take place Sunday, March 28, 2010 during the 11:15 a.m. service at Union Baptist Church. A reception in your honor will follow in the church fellowship hall.

Please meet members of the couples ministry in the front lobby of the church by 10:50 a.m. to be escorted to your reserved seating. You will receive a phone call from Minister Tonetta Killens-Worth shortly with additional information.

Again, congratulations and I look forward to seeing you on March 28.

Sincerely,

Harry Lawson, Chairman
UBC Couples Ministry

# SPIRITUAL COLLISION

Life was good, and my family was moving along fine until a spiritual head on collision brought me to a complete stop. Suddenly traffic shifted and within months of everything moving so fast, I couldn't keep up anymore.

## The Pulpit Transition

I had found a church close to our home in Durham. When I went to visit, it took me back to my old days in Kittrell. The services reminded me of what I loved about church growing up. I knew that God was calling me to join.

After I joined, my whole family followed me in membership. Grear was five when he started ushering and realized it was his ministry. When he joined our new church, that was his service. He continues to usher to this day.

When Bernard was in high school, he became the leader for the youth choir. Nikki became the President of the children's choir, and Clarence sang with the Male Chorus and the Mass Choir. When Grear and Clarence were baptized together, Mother and I were overjoyed.

I attended Sunday school and became one of the Youth Movement advisors for the children. After being there a short time, Pastor came to class one day and said, "Mrs. Yelverton, I want you to be the teacher of the new

Corinthian class." I didn't know what he was talking about and why he was asking me to be an adult Sunday School teacher.

One of the female ministers was standing behind me and she asked, "Can I be your assistant?'

The pastor said, "Teachers' meeting is every Monday night." He turned on his heels and left the classroom. I looked around, but I didn't know what to feel. Everybody started clapping and cheering for me, it felt strange.

When I got home and told Clarence what happened, he was so happy. I was surprised because I knew that his upbringing in the Apostolic faith was similar to the pastor's, in that women were to keep silent. He asked me, "He wants you to be a teacher?" All I could do was shrug my shoulders. I was glad that he supported me.

That Monday night, I went to Teachers' meeting, and Pastor reiterated that he wanted me to teach the Corinthian class. Every Monday, I looked forward to learning how to be a good teacher. To this day, it still warms my heart when my old students remember me. One thing that our pastor taught, that I still carry with me, is how to pray.

In the Corinthians class we lifted our voices every Sunday morning in praise and Thanksgiving. God used me to teach His anointed Word, and I magnified the Holy Spirit.

When the Women's Committee was putting together the plan for Women's Day in 1990, they asked our pastor if I could do the pastoral prayer before his sermon. Some of the teachers felt that I was "an anointed one" for the responsibility (to God be the glory).

Our pastor did not believe that women should be ministers or preachers. For Women's Day, he told us we could ask local motivational speakers or television anchors to address the congregation with a message. We could as well, invite any professional woman, just not a minister.

There were many activities planned for that Sunday in June 1990. I put on my blue dress, ready to pray. Our speaker, also in blue, was a television anchor. I still remember her encouraging message and how kind she was to me.

Waves swept through the congregation that Sunday morning, when I prayed. Nikki was shouting out, "That's my Mama! That's my Mama!"

# FAMILY

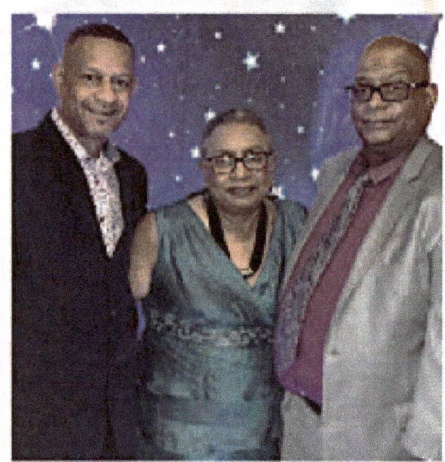

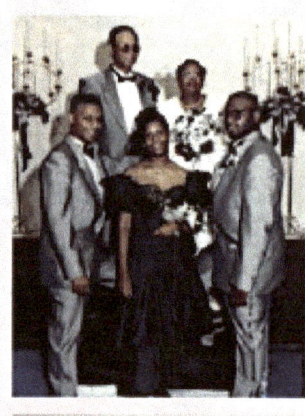

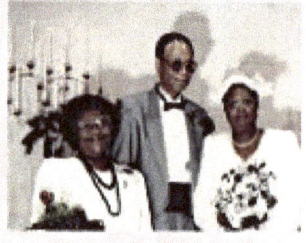

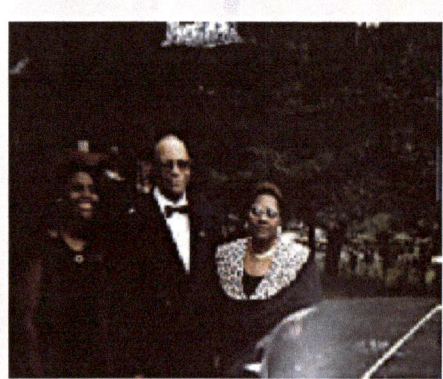

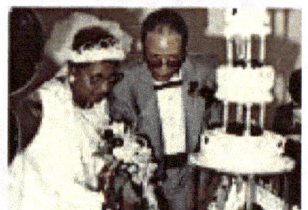

**Pearley's Pearls**
Wisdom From My Journey Through Life

# THE SEIZURE - A HIT AND RUN

On Sunday September 9, 1990, I was rejoicing and praising God. My family was living our best life. Bernard was going to the college of his dreams, and Nikki was entering high school. We had a family trip planned to Florida on September 11, 1990, with our church. On September 10, 1990, my last day before vacation, I had to work a half a day at the hospital. It was Grear's birthday, and I had already sent his gift via UPS, because he had left for the Air Force.

That morning, I was discharging a patient, and she must have noticed some odd movements. She cried out, "Help! Help! There's something wrong with her!" While one rep came and discharged the patient, I was taken to an examination room. The doctors didn't find anything wrong, and I finished my shift.

Let me tell you, God kept me. I left work, got in my car and drove to pick Nikki up from theater rehearsal. When I picked her up she said, "Mom, why are you picking me up early?" I could tell she was upset. "We have a show coming up." I told her we had to get ready for vacation. We went home, microwaved our dinner, showered, and went to bed excited to leave the next day.

Clarence told me later that, I woke him up and went into a grand mal seizure. According to Google, this type of seizure involves violent muscle movements and a loss of consciousness. I fell off of the bed and broke both of my shoulders.

I can explain now what it felt like, when I used to have a seizure. I would see sparkling flickers and watch lights go on and off. My eyes would roll around and around, and I could not think, nor could I speak. Having that seizure, I switched from the "Pulpit of Praise" to the "Prison Walls of Epilepsy."

Can you imagine what would have happened if we had been on the road? God is so good!

My family told me that it took the Emergency Response Team a long while to position my body to get it on the stretcher. It took so long that my sister Beverly and Mother arrived from Franklin County. They drove forty miles and arrived in time to see the ambulance drive away with me. Beverly still talks about seeing the ambulance drive away, knowing that I had had a seizure. It hurt her that she was not able to see me.

Clarence had to break the news to Grear about my seizure. It was hard for Grear. Thankfully, his buddies Sam, Moe, and Terry and the prayers of Saints sustained him through it until he could get home. Grear's friends, the twins, George and Germaine, as well as Bernard's friend Derek, along with our family friend John, held my boys up.

My family stayed in the waiting room waiting for the doctor's report. No one was sleeping, they all just crashed on the floor in the waiting room. If a doctor came into the hall they would ask, "Is there a report for the Yelverton family?"

The physician tried to reply to all of the questions that were asked. He just kept saying, "I will keep you updated should any changes arise, or if we need to change her treatments."

There was no snacking or laughing in the waiting room. My family told me that between other families flipping the TV screen, and the activities on the trauma unit, their anxiety was high. It was as if our happily ever after started falling apart. Clarence was already trying to recover from a heart attack and three months of rehabilitation from triple bypass surgery, and then I got sick, too.

*"Courage is not having the strength to go on; it is going on when you don't have the strength."*

~Teddy Roosevelt

# IS THERE ANY HOPE?

I don't know how many days it took me to wake up, but I was in the ICU when I came to. As I opened my eyes doctors were standing over me. They started firing questions at me:

What is your name?

Do you know where you are?

Who is the President of the United States?

I was able to answer their questions with no problem. One of them told me that I had a seizure. I had a prior seizure after my Toxemia pregnancy; however, the two seizures were unrelated.

Epilepsy is known as abnormal function and activity of the brain, and referred to as Epilepsy Seizure Disorder, if more than two episodes occur within close proximity. Seizures are the most common neurological condition one can have. Everyone with epilepsy has their own story, this is mine.

## My Story of Faith

I was shocked to hear that I had Epilepsy. All I could utter was, "Is there any hope? Does anything matter anymore?" My life was ripped from me, and I was turned upside down. I felt that I had been in a collision with an 18-wheeler, and the driver left the scene. The impact of the spiritual collision after my seizure crushed me in many ways. Again, I needed to lean on the lesson I had learned about perseverance in 4-H Club as a child.

The seizure caused multiple injuries. Both of my shoulders were broken, I lost my vision for a few minutes, my face and lips were swollen, and I had chipped teeth. The big lips that God had given me were much bigger. I looked bad.

Nikki went from shouting with pride, "That's my Mama!" to being traumatized. When she saw me with all of my injuries she asked, "Is that my Mama!?" I was so hurt. Everyone that was in the loop surrounding me was affected by my epilepsy.

The doctors said I was partially paralyzed, but Mother and Aunt Thelma knew I could feel my body. I had memory lapses, too. I couldn't imagine what my family was going through. There were moments I barely knew who I was, or where I was. My face felt abnormal like a helium balloon.

My hospital room walls were overflowing with cards, inspirational books, flowers and balloons. Clarence told me, "People have been talking about your prayer at the Women's Day Service, and how God has moved throughout the Church and the community for the past two days."

Patient Information was giving out my room number before visitors could say my name. The anchorwoman who had spoken at our church attempted to visit me in the hospital, but my family wouldn't allow her in the room. Everyone wanted to protect my privacy because they were afraid that I would end up on the evening news.

One of the surgeons said, "I have never seen so much love in a hospital room." He reached down to pick up some cards that had fallen and tried to tape them back on the door. It gave my cousin an idea for how to rearrange them for the time.

The next morning a grouchy interim doctor came through the same door saying, "You need to get some of this stuff out the way."

"How unthoughtful of him," I thought. I was lying there with two broken shoulders.

No one would allow me to see myself. I kept asking for a mirror, but my family wouldn't give me one. I saw a friend coming down the hall, and I called him into my room. When he saw me he looked shocked. I asked him, "Would you please go to the gift shop and get me a mirror?"

When he came back with the mirror, and I saw myself, I felt like a monster. I saw my broken shoulders, the cast and a sling. I was not normal anymore; I was in so much excruciating pain. I didn't have a clue of how to go forward. I was comforted that Mother was there with me most of the time.

It was traumatic for Clarence and the children after my seizure. Bernard and Nikki saw me on a daily basis. Bernard had transferred from Virginia Union to North Carolina Central because he needed to be on dialysis. He was able to receive treatment and prepare for a transplant while being able to support me, since

Grear was not able to be there. Everything was going in different directions. I was trying to cling to my hope.

It crushed Bernard when we had to bring him home after his first semester. We loved him, and the doctor said, "Bring him home." The pearl of wisdom I got from that moment is that you never know hurt and disappointment until it knocks on your door. It was five years of misery before finding a match for him, but God did it!

Eventually, Clarence had to go back to work, and the children went back to school. God continued to elevate him on his job, and he asked me not to return to work when he said, "Pudding, I got this." I was so grateful my Boo was so caring; however, I needed a sense of self-worthiness, and the courage to be true to myself. I yearned for something to give me the chance to move forward from this difficult circumstance, and I thought about volunteering.

## The After Effects of Epilepsy

Life was passing me by. I had to dispel the anguish, grumbling and disappointment in order to reboot myself. The reboot happened, and I came back swinging. Through the gaps and pauses of life's circumstances, God taught me what is and what isn't important. I know that my life matters to God.

My faith was dwindling with all of the unsuccessful treatments. My quality of life seemed to have bottomed out, as I laid motionless between hope and shoulder slings. My memory still had not healed. They couldn't do reconstructive surgery for over a year, because my right shoulder was where the breast cancer had been. Swelling in that arm could have caused other complications for me.

## Treatments

Doctor Vann tried to bring me down off the high doses of Dilantin because my feet were becoming numb. He said, "You have a choice Pearley, seizures or neuropathy." He gave me a new medication; after the breakthrough of seven consecutive seizures, I was in a critical stage.

I needed to take a good look at my life and recognize Thanksgiving and praise, even in this storm. I needed to learn to appreciate the joy and the beauty of all of the blessings in my life. Today, I have to be eternally grateful for the things I once took for granted, like researching for medication. Years ago, Barbital was the only medicine around for long-term pain management and it just kept you asleep most of the time. Thank God there are so many new medications.

I was on so much medication; I used to fall asleep standing up sometimes. Trying to maintain my independence, I went to deposit some money into the bank and fell asleep in the line while holding my deposit slip. People were walking past me and no one helped. Grear finally came in to see what was taking me so long. I can't count how many times I was accused of being intoxicated. People just don't understand the side effects of epilepsy medication.

### "Them Old Thangs"

Back in the day, active seizures were called, "fits," or "them old thangs." That's what Mother and Ms. Emery, my ninety-three-year-old neighbor, across the street, used to call them. In our neighborhood, Clarence and I were the first Black family. We met Ms. Emery and her daughter, Jackie, when we moved in, but her husband didn't speak to us.

When I had my seizure, and they heard the fire truck and ambulance, Ms. Emery and her daughter Jackie came across the street to see what was happening. Clarence told her and her daughter that he didn't know what was happening. He was glad that they stayed with him for a while.

For several months, when I would have a seizure, Clarence would call the EMS. Jackie would say, "You know Mama loves Mrs. Pearley." Ms. Emery would be so worried, she would say, "I hope Pearley is alright, and not having one of them old thangs."

One particular morning, the doorbell rang, and it was Jackie. She said, "You know how Mama feels about you. She had to go in that kitchen and cook up somethin'." My mouth was so sore that I couldn't eat the pie she made. Clarence called to thank them, and he mentioned that it was my birthday. Ms. Emery made chicken and dumplings and the biggest apple pie I've ever seen, all from scratch.

After I had a seizure, Ms. Emery used to call me and say, "How you feeling baby? I prayed last night for you to be alright when I heard that EMS and that siren."

When I felt up to it, Bernard would walk me across the street to visit with her.

One day, Jackie invited some Sunday School teachers and a few of her other friends to come fellowship with us. When we were together, she never knew I heard her whisper, "Be nice to her. She is a nice colored girl with a nice family."

Ms. Emery was my friend, and I loved her. She taught me about acceptance. From the day we moved into her neighborhood in Durham, she welcomed our family to church, community activities and Watch Care services. Her kindness and care will never be forgotten.

*"Hope is being able to see that there is light despite all of the darkness."*

~Desmond Tutu

# THERE IS HOPE

I joined UBC in 2000; I was drawn back there. I had fond memories of my first job there. One morning in 2002, after 7:30 morning worship services, I was driving Clarence to his Apostolic church in Rocky Mount, North Carolina. I was sleepy, but I was trying to hold it all together. I blinked and ended up in another city. Oh yes, I have been in the valley of the shadow of death. It was terrible, believe me.

Thanks be to God I didn't crash. Someone bigger than me snatched me back, woke me up, and I continued the drive on that country road. I had to stop to get some black coffee.

When Clarence talked about it later, I asked him why he didn't say something. He replied, "It wasn't talking time, it was praying time."

Finally, I got a breakthrough when a big giant orange pill was approved in March 2000 for Epilepsy treatments. My doctor gave me the prescription before it hit the market. Because of him, my local drug store investigated it and ordered it.

The Bible says, "They that wait upon the Lord shall renew their strength. They shall mount up on wings like eagles." Paul said, "When I was weak I was strong."

The impact of that spiritual collision (my seizure) was so intense it took me twelve years to recover from it. After eleven and one half years of suffering, I finally made it to six months without a seizure because of the new medication. It's been more than twenty-two years since I had my first seizure, and I can't help but thank God for healing me and allowing me to drive a car again.

Since my diagnosis, I have been my own advocate trying to reconnect with life in spite of epilepsy. I was so terrified, I didn't want to talk about it to anyone. For twenty-two years, I battled breast cancer and epilepsy, but having epilepsy has caused me to have a complex heart condition. It was my worst pitfall.

In 1992, I had to have reparative surgery for my shoulders. During that surgery I had a heart attack that required another surgery. I have experienced shame and I know what it feels like to live behind a prison wall called the "Fear of the Unknown."

But God!

In 2000, I had surgery to implant a device under my skin called Vagus Nerve Stimulation (VNS). I was one of the first people to receive this innovative surgery. This therapy helps control my seizures. I call the machine my "engine," because it vibrates on the left side of my chest twenty-four hours a day. My VNS allows me to move in a new direction, and reach far beyond feeling well. If I accidentally tap the button, it will alert an operator who will say, "Triangle Life Line, Mrs. Yelverton are you alright?"

My family had a reception for me, when I reached six months of being seizure free. After twelve years of uncontrolled seizures, the VNS was a life changer. It allowed me to switch out of that slow-moving lane of hopelessness.

## Durham Epilepsy Support Team

How do you spell relief? Support. Support. Support. There is strength in changing lives one day at a time. Like the African Proverb says, "Each one reach one," our purpose is to raise awareness about epilepsy and be a beacon of light to those who suffer daily with this disorder. Our mission is to educate the public and bring down the stigma and misconceptions of epilepsy. Our team's foundation is built on Proverbs 17:22: "*A merry heart is like medicine, but the crushed spirit dries up the bones.*"

I became a member of the Durham Mayor's Committee for Persons with Disabilities in 2007. Pat Gibson, my Director from the Carolina Epilepsy Alliance of North Carolina, North Carolina Senator Mike Woodard, and US Congressman David Price are such gems to me. The former mayor of Durham, William Bell, and Cora Cole-McFadden, the Mayor Pro Tempore, allowed me to host an Epilepsy walk in Durham. Mayor Bell signed the first Proclamation for an Annual Epilepsy Awareness Month.

Many thanks are in order to Ken and Gwen who contributed much into our group. They demonstrated what multiplied team efforts can produce. It is fitting that they lifted the opening logo for Durham First's Epilepsy Fall 5K Fall Stroll. Our theme that year was, "Every Stroll Opens a new Path for Epilepsy."

Having epilepsy has allowed me to walk through doors of opportunities I otherwise wouldn't have had. I was an Emeritus Board Member of North Carolina Epilepsy Foundation. I'm the co-founder, and I have been the team chair for the Durham Epilepsy support team for over twenty years. Being a member of this diverse committee is part of my mission to reach back and lift others. It provides me with valuable resources and opportunities for people with disabilities.

Mother didn't want me to go public with my epilepsy diagnosis, yet she cheered for me and supported me in private. She was excited when she received her first receipt for a contribution to The North Carolina Epilepsy Foundation. They hymn she used to sing, "Steal Away" at Haywood Baptist Church has brought me joy throughout my journey. Mother died on September 11, 2007. Losing her made me feel like my twin towers had fallen. I was grateful when my family told me that the Epilepsy Stroll was dedicated to her in 2007. Her light will forever shine in Durham Epilepsy.

Clarence was standing by Mother's casket in Louisburg, North Carolina when he saw a bright shining light. We saw a miracle when God restored his vision. It was a Thursday night when Clarence woke up screaming, "Pudding! Pudding where are you? I can't see you." We didn't know it, but Clarence had a stroke and lost his sight. We had known for a while he was legally blind, and we prayed without ceasing for healing. I am grateful for many things, including his restored vision. And, it's been twenty-two years, and I can't help but thank God for healing me.

# LOSING MY DRIVING PRIVILEGES

One Monday when she was sixteen, I was driving Nikki to work because she was late. She was a brand new driver, and I was nervous about her driving on the highway. Driving along, she talked to me about her friend, and I went into a seizure. A bread truck was behind me blowing his horn and other drivers were putting their middle fingers up, screaming and shouting at me.

Nikki said, "Somehow, some way, God gave me supernatural strength to move the car." She said that 18-wheelers were flying by her so fast that she could feel the wind from them. God gave her the power to push the car off of the bypass from Highway 85 to a grassy area. She walked up the hill to a service station to call my son Grear.

When the police officer arrived, I was coming to from the seizure. He said, I am going write on the ticket that you had a stroke."

"Why?" I asked.

"If I write that you had a seizure, they will revoke your license." I knew it was the right thing to do, and it took twelve years before I could drive again.

## My Independence Day

I know we celebrate July 4th as Independence Day, but I also celebrate March 16, when I received my letter from North Carolina Division of Motor Vehicles with my photo license. I was grateful for the taxi cab vouchers I'd received from my former employer, Duke Medical Center that allowed me to be able to get back and forth; however, I also thought about how Clarence bought me a burgundy Buick and parked it in the yard. He wanted me to see it every day and be inspired to drive again. Oh what a giant of faith he saw in me.

I realize success isn't always titles and positions or the routes you travel. It is the struggles you endure and overcome to reach your destiny. As it turns out, I learned that my license had actually been revoked, but it was for the right reasons—I had epilepsy. Dr. Vann went in the waiting room and said to Bernard, "After twelve years of active seizures, your Mom is six-months seizure-free."

I called it blessed. He came back and said to me, "You can prepare for your driver's license. Go to the DMV, pick up a manual and read every word before you take the test."

## Released to Drive

Before my driving privileges were revoked, I had been driving for twenty-five years. The system may not have changed much but, it was certainly challenging getting them back in to swing. I was so excited about getting my License.

I was given a day in court to determine if I could drive again. It was a divine appointment from the moment we hit the grounds. I can't describe what I was feeling that day. I didn't have a clue about this judge who was assigned to me, but we saw him outside of the building. It was obvious he wasn't ready. He didn't have on his black robe; he wasn't carrying a brief case, and his papers were flying all over the ground. The wind was so strong whipping in every direction, we had to hold our coats closed.

Grear, being the person that he is, rushed out of the car and began running to chase the folders. The scene reminded me of Hurricane Hazel. Grear picked up what he could and gave them to the man. It seemed that gratitude was not part of his vocabulary. When we entered the building, the receptionist received us with kindness. As we waited, we heard the Judge calling for His first case. The receptionist said, "Go right on in Mrs. Yelverton." Grear followed me into the room.

The judge looked at us over his glasses. We recognized each other, and he was just as cold as he had been outside. I became anxious as he began asking questions about a stroke. Grace and mercy kicked in and turned up the heat. Grear began to speak for me. He said, "Your Honor, my mother has epilepsy."

I found out two weeks later that the judge had granted me my driving privileges. Once I showed him the note from my doctor, I thought about how Nikki and my granddaughter, Jordyn, used to say, "Yes, you can," when I didn't think I could drive again. I was so happy when I could drive again. The first time I drove with Jordyn in the car, she reached for my hand from her booster seat and said, "Grandma, we need to pray." Her little heart was so sweet.

## Do Not Quit

One particular day, I was trying to find some peace so I drove around to clear my head. I ended up stopping at Jordyn's school during their thirty minute fun time. We exchanged hugs and kisses that overflowed; we were so happy to see other. I had to hold back my tears, because I was everyone's Grandma for the moment.

I sat with Jordyn and watched as the other children played. Ninety five percent of them were sharing dolls, stuffed animals or action figures. Jordyn grabbed some building blocks. She was concentrating as she stacked them, and when her tower got too high, they would fall.

I watched her rebuild the tower so many times that I lost count. It seemed that she got more excited each time the tower fell. She would shout, "Grandma! Grandma! Look!" The blocks were so unstable that a sneeze could have knocked them over. Jordyn didn't care, every time her tower would fall, she built it higher the next time.

For a minute, I was distracted from my life's disappointments, as I sat in the classroom with the happy children. When I left the school, I was inspired by Jordyn's perseverance and determination not to quit when building her tower. She found a way to build a skyscraper that pleased her. Jordyn and her classmates reminded me not to let life knock me down! Arriving home, I took out my Handicap Placard ready to accept the things I could not change.

Once I started driving again, I didn't know about the changes to the driving laws in North Carolina. I expected some things to be different, but I was shocked one day when I received a long white envelope with a fifty dollar ticket from the Quick Pass Toll. A photo of my license plate was included, because I had exceeded the speed limit without having a clue.

Eventually driving became natural for me again.

.

# THE WHOLE PERSON

**Please be at ease**
**If you are in close proximity of a person**
**with epilepsy or a disability**
**Either visible or hidden.**

**Believe me, you share the same air**
**They laugh, they play and they work.**

**If you reach deep inside of your hearts**
**If you are willing**
**To appreciate them for their culture**
**Qualites and lucrative contributioms**
**that they give**
**Perhaps then you would**
**see the whole person.**
~Pearley Long Yelverton, Epilepsy Warrior

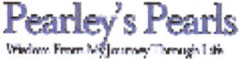
Pearley's Pearls
Wisdom From My Journey Through Life

# A SEASON OF GRIEF

When Clarence was sick, I chose to volunteer at the hospital on the heart unit. That way, I was close to him, yet I could serve other people.

I felt so good giving back. I always wanted to stay connected to the elderly, and I was profoundly motivated to aid people who are visually impaired.

Volunteering was a pleasure and after my Epilepsy diagnosis, it was more than enough to keep me motivated. I didn't mind when Clarence told one of his elderly coworkers that I would come fry fish for him, his twin brother, and his wife. They were all visually impaired. Mildred, the wife, knew how to cook, but she didn't feel comfortable frying anything on the stove because of her blindness. I went over their house and cooked. They enjoyed the food, and I enjoyed serving it to them.

My pastor was encouraging the congregation to get involved with services in our community. Pastor Hammond invited a volunteer minister to speak to the church. In his message that Sunday he said, "When all you have is nothing, nothing is enough." That reminded me of our fire when I was a child. I was grateful for what I had.

## My Boo Slipped Away

My beloved passed away on June 19, 2014. During his illness and hospice care, my family became strength and courage for me. Clarence had suffered four heart attacks, coronary bypass surgery and coronary stents. Even though he was ill, Clarence never lost his faith. We were active in our church and served others whenever we could.

When he was in the hospital during his last days, my brother-in-law, Michael sat at his feet quietly, shushing everyone and admonishing them to be quiet. Each time my sister, Beverly entered she brought something she thought would make him comfortable. My sister, Carolyn checked the nurses' time sheets. Our family friends, Kim and Marisa, brought dinner each Sunday while Pastor Linda Harris knelt at his feet in prayer. Cousin Deborah sat with him on Thursdays. Cousin Linda went with me and sat with us during Respite Care.

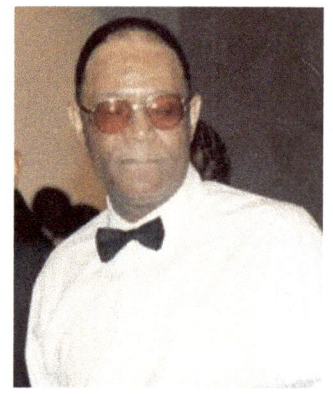

One evening I left the hospital because I needed to go home, shower, and tidy up the house. I wanted to lie down for a short nap in my own bed. As I dozed I could feel Clarence's heartbeat. Grear came to my bedroom door and said, "Nikki called and said come back." In that moment of stillness, while Beverly, Micheal and Kim watched over him, my Boo slipped away. He was seventy-six.

When I arrived back at the hospital, Nikki courageously swung the door open, but her body language showed me that something was wrong. My heart thumped in my chest. "Clarence, why didn't you wait for me?" I thought as tears filled my eyes.

Losing my husband slowed my wheels, and I became immobilized. In the midst of family, feuds, and rejections, I was lonely. God was with me, but my family chain was broken. Nothing has been the same, since Clarence slipped away. When God calls us home one by one, our chains will link again. I know Clarence will always be with me, yet not seeing him in his favorite seat really hurts me sometimes.

When Clarence transitioned to his eternal home, I moved into Widow's Lane. My foundation was becoming fragile, and his absence was evident. The pillows were not enough to hold on to, but I clutched them. Holding on to them allowed me to clutch those precious memories of my Boo.

**Widow's Lane**

Rev. Dr. Kenneth Ray Hammond and his wife, First Lady Evelyn, were so compassionate with us, after my husband died. Their flowing of the written word for my husband's Homegoing Celebration moved me. The title of his eulogy, "I Can See Clearly Now," will always reinstate my faith if I am feeling down.

My dear friend Francis didn't have the funds to travel to Clarence's funeral but she raised the money to come by playing the lottery. I was so happy that she made the sacrifice to be there for me. Another friend drove to Kittrell, from Fayetteville, to pick up one of our mutual friends. After the funeral, she drove her back to Durham and back to Kittrell. That was so kind.

I heard others say in Grief Counseling that their families and friends neglected them after the loss of their spouse. I didn't think that would ever happen to me. But it did. Clarence and I had shared our hearts and home with so many people. Shortly after he was gone, some of those relationships waxed cold. Many times I felt like a misfit after he died. No one rang the doorbell other than FedEx, UPS and the Saturday morning Witnesses.

After losing Clarence, I was back at a crossroad. I was waiting for the light to change, giving me permission to move forward. I realized that I had moved to a new lane. Clarence will always be in the passenger seat in my heart, but I have to ride it out alone now.

My Divine Healer spoke to me during that time. When I was at that gloomiest hour of my life, God brought His glory. He embraced me with His loving arms and whispered in my ear, "I want you to follow your dreams. I am going to throw you a party, and I am picking up the tab. Pearley, I want you to revamp, revitalize and resume your writing journey."

## Living Beyond The Loss

On Widow's Lane, I had to be more aware of the caution lights, speed bumps and roundabouts on my journey. After a friend's party one night, I was left on an old dark deserted highway country road, alone with my car. There were four drivers in the other car and nothing around me other than trees, trees, and more trees. Somehow I found my way back home.

I learned that night to recognize that everyone grieves differently. Through it all, I learned to move beyond the crossroad of my own grief. From my experience, I wrote and submitted a proposal to my pastor to create a program that would support families in their grief to live beyond the loss. I called the group, "Living Beyond The Loss."

### Living Beyond the Loss

"We all have heard that time heals all wounds but these last 16 months for me have been very difficult.

Grieving has reminded me as a child building my block bridge; every time I think I got it licked there I see a little side leaning.

As an adult London Bridge come tumbling down the hill like a spring time down pour.

·  Recent Widow

*Proposal:* Living Beyond Loss (LBL) Unity Team

*Purpose:* While this is not a Support Group, to be mindful, thoughtful and most of all prayerful for those who are ready for the outreach, in dealing with the loss of a Spouse, to know they are not alone and can find some joy.

*Approach:* Although we know we never can fill the void, we can offer:

+ A phone call to say, "I was thinking about you today."
+ A hug.
+ A card, thoughtful note or Email.
+ A visit.

Each One
Reach one

*Goals:* Empower those Bereaved to learn ways, means and strategies to embrace the real world in their new setting and build relationships.

*Events:* With consideration being given to busy schedules we can eat, talk and be merry over:

+ Breakfast
+ Brunch
+ Lunch
+ Dinner

*Communication:* Be mindful not to consume anyone.

+ Email
+ Telephone
+ Postal Mail
+ Visit telephone, or visit email

We hope all will find healing and a safe place In the words of the Serenity Prayer below:

God, grant me the Serenity

To accept the things

I cannot change...

The Courage to change the things I can,

And the Wisdom to know the difference

·

Humbly Submitted

Paisley Long/Stamm

Slogan

96

Here I stand at the altar of Union Baptist, which is my safe place. The symbol of the cross comforts me. These memorial flowers were for my beloved husband. My restoration begins at the cross.

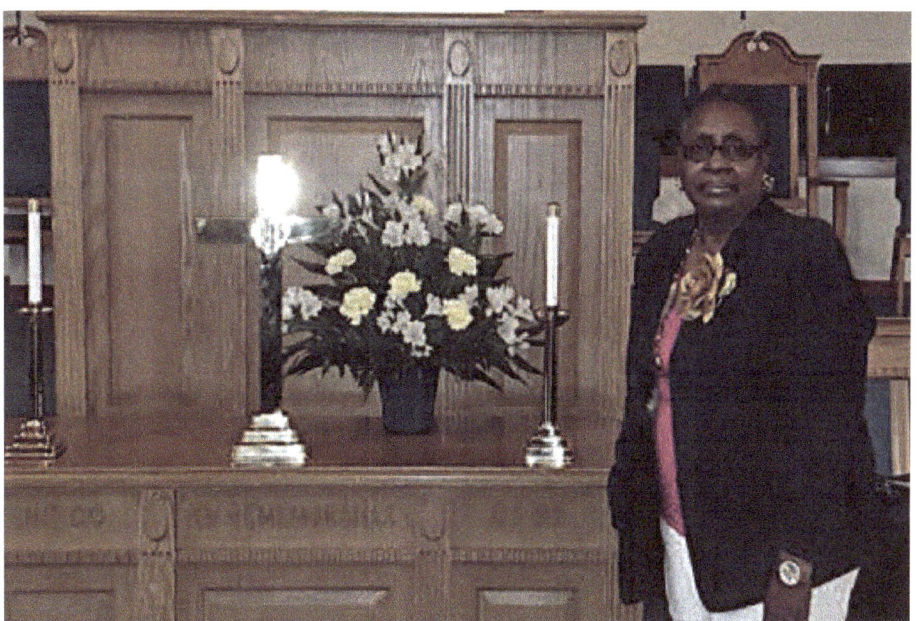

*"Through the grace of God, I deem it's my time to shine!"*

~Pearley Long Yelverton

# LIFE IS A BLESSING

My life has been a journey that has taken me through many roads and detours. With my breastplate of righteousness, having girded my lions, I have been able to stand against the schemes of the enemy along the highway of life. The first thing I do every day is put on the whole armor of God.

Along my journey, God has shown me the light, and I have picked up pearls of wisdom. Oh Lord, when I think about my journey and how He placed angels to watch over me, I let the praise begin from the bottom of my heart. Despite all the frustrations, setbacks, gaps, even throwing in the hat several times, I buckled down, set boundaries, and quarantined with God to get instructions to pursue my goals.

Even though I didn't finish college, one of my greatest accomplishments was volunteering at an elementary School in Henderson, North Carolina. They named me as an honorary principal that day.

I have been truly tested and have developed unwavering faith even running on empty. When I felt isolated, God reached into the depths of my soul. As the wheels of my faith journey turned, it didn't matter what line of traffic or how intense the flow, I remained focused and kept going. I knew it was a fork in the road, and my help was right around the bend. I had to keep pushing through life's construction sites, even when I wanted to take a glimpse at the peak of the landslide.

"Amazing Grace" will always be my song of praise. God lifted me, kept me, and guided me through daily challenges. Some have heard it, some have sung it, some have talked it . . . I have lived it. My soul cries out "Hallelujah!" My hope is built on nothing less, than Jesus's Blood and His righteousness, as the song says. While I may be hearing impaired, I can always hear my Father talking. My spirit continues to hear one of my favorite Baptist Hymns, "Draw me Nearer."

It was Amazing Grace that allowed me to stay focused on my purpose. Even when I threw in the hat, something inside kept telling me, "Stay with it, never give up. I've got you." Through every season His mercy endures forever. Be encouraged, when God's got you, He's got you.

God has allowed me to see, on my journey, that He has always been with me. Take this pearl of wisdom and tuck it in your heart: look at what God has put before you every day and thank Him for the journey. Let praise time be all the time, because He is always there.

I want you to think about the gloomiest time in your life. Take the time to dig deep inside and remember how you made it through that difficult time. Connect with the essence of your soul where only you and your Greater One dwell. Do a full system scan of your life and wait for the results. We can't say our engines are fully operational right now, but we can always say we have a Master Mechanic to care for every need we have.

Through the grace of God, I deem it's my time to shine! I will not allow my vulnerabilities and apprehensions to become my master again. God not only added years to my life, but life to my years. He will do the same for you. Jesus was the center of my joy, I didn't just survive, I thrived. My fringe benefits were the greatest salary I ever received. Only God knows how I felt when I was finally washed in the precious blood of the Lamb and got my life back.

I will never forget the topic of a speaker who came to UBC's Back-to-School Breakfast for Youth Church. She was a member of our church and an attorney. Her message was, 'You got the Keys." I thought about her message and all the things God has brought me through. I was reminded of how many times the Greater One has snatched me back into His arms and put me back together. Sometimes I feel like I am flying, without wings, with the Divine Navigator who knows the way.

When I was in the valley, I was able to get a good snapshot of Him. In the dark rooms, God was developing me like a piece of film so He could create the real image of me. Through fasting and praying, I'm on the big screen with my Master.

It's time for you to gather your pearls.

Pearley

# LET
# PRAISE
# TIME
# BEGIN!

Pearley's Pearls
Wisdom From My Journey Through Life

# NEWSPAPER
# CLIPPINGS

## Breast cancer survivor inspires 'gem' of activism

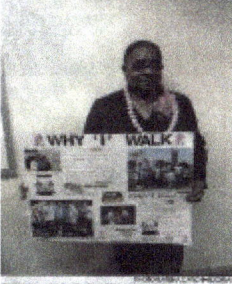

## Breast cancer survivor inspires 'gem' of an organization

By Latisha Catchatoorian

DURHAM — Pearley Long Yelverton's son refers to her as the "gem of the sea," and through her advocacy of breast cancer awareness, she's has been a jewel.

As a 38-year survivor, Yelverton has dedicated the last three decades to breast cancer awareness. Though October is breast cancer awareness month, it is clear by her breast cancer ribbon-printed cellphone case and the pink flower she wears on her lapel, that the disease stays on her mind all year round.

At the 2012 Susan G. Komen Race for the Cure, Yelverton was announced as the longest breast cancer survivor in Durham. She was diagnosed in July 1976 and had a mastectomy and 16 lymph nodes removed. She also endured 18 months of chemotherapy.

"It was the most numbing thing I've ever heard. It was disbelief; it was numbness. My husband and my children were truly survivors also, because my baby was 18 months old (at the time.) My whole life turned around because I was 29 years old," she said. "When you hear the word cancer, the first thing you think about is dying. That was my prayer, that I would see my children grown."

Yelverton, who had three young

Please see BREAST/3A

## Pearley's Pearls
Wisdom From My Journey Through Life

# PEARLS OF WISDOM

### Rule 1:
Never give up on your dreams.

### Rule 2:
Be in it to win it.

### Rule 3:
Be in it to win it.

### Rule 4:
Sometimes life takes you down in
order to bring you back even better
than before

### Rule 5:
Never give up on Rule 1.

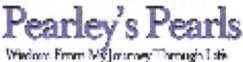

Pearley's Pearls
Wisdom From My Journey Through Life

# EPILOGUE
## LET THE PRAISE TIME BEGIN

*I have been afflicted that I may learn your statues.*
Psalm 119:71 (NKJV)

God has exhibited, in my journey, a multitude of miraculous acts. Here are some additional praise reports and testimonies from my life that I want to share with you. I hope they encourage you:

### Ignored by the Priest

In January of 2003, I had to have surgery to repair my knee. I tripped over a plastic mat in my daughter's room and hurt my knee and ankle. After being in the hospital for seven days, I had to go to a nursing home to recover and have extensive physical therapy. That Good Friday, a priest came to pray for my roommate. They asked if I wanted prayer, and he did not respond.

Behind his back, the other resident and their family asked if I wanted prayer. They said it loud enough for him to hear, and he still didn't respond. Behind his back, they blew me kisses. It was fine with me that he didn't ask; I had a loving pastor. I could tell that they were hurt by his lack of attention, and when he left, they shared their palms with me.

One morning, during a physical therapy session, two staff members came over to assist me and some other patients with getting out of the pool before our session was over. We all were confused because our therapy had just begun. I asked, "What is happening?"

One of the staff members said, "We are closing the pool, it is disconnecting from the wall, but the specialist is coming." I thought to myself, "Jesus is the only water specialist I know!"

## Stuck on a Train Track

One night I was in overdrive, leaving the hospital where my son was, and I was trying to get to my Aunt Thelma who had surgery. I was so distraught; I drove right under a train track arm. The arms of the track were flapping up and down, but did not touch the hood of my car. I was blowing and trying to get the car behind me to move but it wouldn't.

Words failed me, and I was numb. I couldn't even utter a one word prayer, "Jesus."

As I sat there, a tape began to rewind to my childhood. I remembered a train tragedy with three fatalities. A family of four was in the car, one person survived. I thought about my uncle telling me, "If there is ever a crisis, call the prayer band. I mustered the strength to pray, and God allowed me to move my car.

## Feeling Alone

One day I was standing in the Walmart parking lot, talking with a friend, when I had a seizure. Nikki was with me, and she was talking with my friend's daughters. When I went down from my seizure, the lady grabbed her daughters' hands and ran across the parking lot.

I can imagine how seeing someone having a seizure can be frightening, but I didn't understand why she left my little girl alone on the curbside. God prevailed, and Nikki found a phone to call Grear. He came and took us home, leaving my car there until I felt better to drive it home.

## Flying to Wisconsin

When my sister Carolyn graduated from college in 1974, I took my first airplane ride to Madison, Wisconsin. Very soon after takeoff, a quiet voice came on the loudspeaker, "May we have your attention please. We are running into some turbulence. The pilots are doing everything they can to resolve this issue."

They told us to remain calm, but I was worried. "Pearley, what have you gotten yourself into?" I thought. "You left your whole family, and here you are above the clouds with turbulence." How was I supposed to remain calm?

Eventually, we made it out of the turbulence and arrived safely.

## God's Resuscitation

God's heart machine kept me and my heart in the right rhythm, even when a machine said, I was brain dead. After a seizure, I was in the hospital recuperating. I was awakened when I heard the neurology team enter my room. A voice I didn't recognize said, "She is brain dead." They never spoke my name. A doctor checked me again and said, "The monitoring equipment was malfunctioning. She is alive. Pearley is alive!"

I want you to know that this is an example of how God has never left my side!

## Wisdom From Mother

When I was younger, Mother encouraged me so much. She told me about a time when she went to the post office. She tapped the glue to put on her stamp for an envelope, and the glue poured out. "That's how I see you after each pitfall. Pearley, you just kept on flowing."

I passed that inspiration to my daughter, Nikki. During my illness and uncertainty, my daughter earned a crown for Miss Black North Carolina, in 1995. I stood with her and tried to get back in the swing of things as she toured with the Honorable James B. Hunt, Jr., North Carolina's Governor.

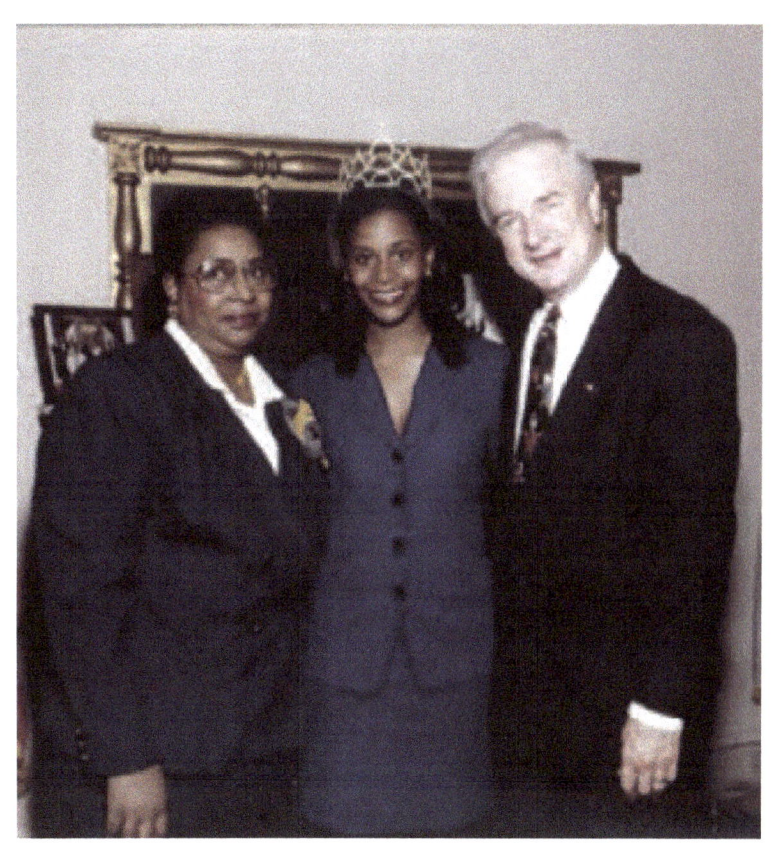

## Pseudo Tumor Cerebra

Of course it was scary when the eye specialist led me to believe something might be wrong. I was not released from a morning appointment at 9:00 to attend a 3:00 afternoon appointment.

At 3:15, I was still sitting in the waiting room hoping for answers. I said to the nurse, "I need to pick up my children and my husband." They knew our family. By this time, I was crying, and she hugged me with tears in her eyes.

The nurse said, "Wait a moment," and left me sitting there. I had no idea what was going on.

When I arrived home, I called the doctor, and he told me he was concerned about the floaters in my eyes, "Mainly about the raised pressure behind your optic nerve." Every month they had to go into my spine to release the fluid. I was still on chemo recovery for breast cancer. The doctor said, "Mrs. Yelverton I want you to go directly to the hospital. They are waiting for you." He made reservations for me to be admitted for further testing. "I am concerned, and I need to know if you have a brain tumor or if your breast cancer is metastatic. I truly was trying to hold it all together.

My sister wanted to go for coffee and a cigarette. I was reluctant and explained what they said. She replied, "If they think you have a brain tumor, a cigarette and coffee aren't going to hurt you."

Two days later, at 1:30, on Sunday morning, the doctor came into my room and said, "I have good and bad news." He confirmed that I had a Pseudotumor Cerebri, meaning there was edema behind the optic nerve. The symptoms were headache, dizziness and possible vision loss. I had floaters across my eyes which was my original reason for going to the optometrist. I didn't need surgery, but treatments included monthly painful spinal injections to release the edema off my optic nerve.

I remember the scripture Jesus spoke about taking the sting out of physical death. It still hurt, but knowing God was at work through such a caring medical staff made it easier. It continued for more than a year, until they got the edema under control. By this time, the seizures were conflicting. Sometimes my family had no idea the things I had to endure.

I was truly suffering with multiple illnesses, but I had to come to a place of acceptance then take option one or two. I had to decide to stop throwing pity parties. I wanted to be healed. I can't tell you what happened. I was transferred to another neurologist, and somehow the headache and floaters all went away.

Let the praise time begin!

# ABOUT THE AUTHOR

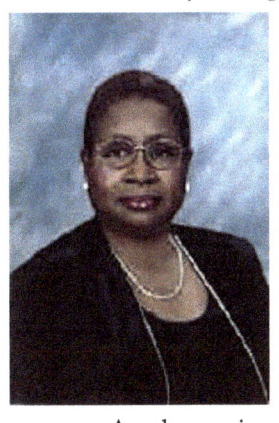 Pearley Long Yelverton was born and raised in Kittrell, North Carolina, as the middle child and oldest daughter of Joe and Sallie Long. Her foundation of faith, service, athleticism, and hard work was formed at an early age. She and her siblings worked on their farm, participated in 4-H Club and attended Sunday school.

A long-time resident of Durham, North Carolina, "The Bull City," Pearley is an advocate and supporter for women living with chronic illnesses. She has been a breast cancer survivor for more than forty-nine years. Her awards include the "More Than Pink Award," given at the Triangle Race For The Cure, in 2019. Pearley was honored with the North Carolina Ruth Bowen Founder's Award, the Epilepsy Foundation of North Carolina Distinguished Service Award, and Who's Who Among Cambridge VIP. Her work experience in Duke Medicine's Financial Management spanned thirty-four years, before she retired.

Pearley is a board member of the Durham Mayor's Committee for Persons with Disabilities, and her proudest moment was being selected as Honorary Principal for Vance County Elementary School.

Pearley has been a member of the historic Union Baptist Church, in Durham, for many years. Her involvement in Disciple Intake, Caregivers, Breast Cancer Support, and Epilepsy Support Ministries is her service to God. She and her late husband, Clarence, were married for over forty years before he passed. She and her "Boo" bore four children, Clarence Jr., Grear, Bernard, and Nikki. Pearly is the proud grandmother of Jordyn Pennie Yelverton.

A writer since childhood, Pearley's works include: *My Epilepsy Hero, A Prep Course for New Parents, Who's That's Lady?, Is There Any Hope?, and The Blood. Pearley's Pearls* is her first publication.